Lifestyle-Related Diseases and Metabolic Syndrome

Edited by Naofumi Shiomi

Published in London, United Kingdom

Lifestyle-Related Diseases and Metabolic Syndrome
http://dx.doi.org/10.5772/intechopen.100992
Edited by Naofumi Shiomi

Contributors
Masayo Nagai, Claudia Andrea Carvallo, Mohammed Ibrahim Sadik, Kotsedi Daniel Monyeki, James Hlengani Siweya, Phut Johanna Makgae, Sarvesh Sabarathinam, Rajappan Chandra Satish Kumar, Thangavel Mahalingam Vijayakumar, Mohammed Abdu, Diress Mengistie, Yonas Akalu, Baye Dagnew Mekonnon, Abdelilah Arredouani, António Gerson Bastos Francisco, Henrique Cotchi Simbo Muela, Amílcar Bernardo Tomé da Silva, Isaura da Conceição Almeida Lopes, Naofumi Shiomi

First published in London, United Kingdom, 2022 by IntechOpen
IntechOpen is the global imprint of INTECHOPEN LIMITED, registered in England and Wales, registration number: 11086078, 5 Princes Gate Court, London, SW7 2QJ, United Kingdom

British Library Cataloguing-in-Publication Data
A catalogue record for this book is available from the British Library

Additional hard and PDF copies can be obtained from orders@intechopen.com

Lifestyle-Related Diseases and Metabolic Syndrome
Edited by Naofumi Shiomi
p. cm.
Print ISBN 978-1-80356-779-2
Online ISBN 978-1-80356-780-8
eBook (PDF) ISBN 978-1-80356-781-5

Meet the editor

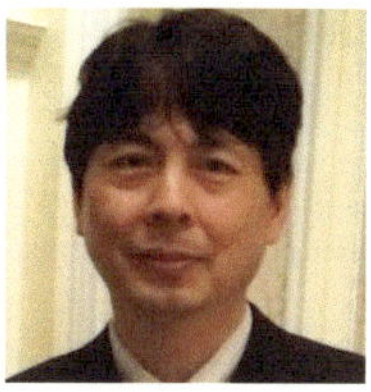

Naofumi Shiomi is a professor at the School of Human Sciences at Kobe College, Japan, where he teaches applied microbiology, biotechnology, and life science. He earned his Ph.D. in engineering from Kyoto University. He studied recombinant yeast and its utilization as a researcher at the Laboratory of Production Technology of Kaneka Corporation for 15 years, and for the last 20 years has studied bioremediation at Kobe College. During the last decade, his research has focused on cellular rejuvenation and the prevention of metabolic syndrome.

Contents

Preface

Lifestyle-related diseases, such as type 2 diabetes, heart disease, and hypertension, are caused by an unbalanced diet and irregular, undesirable lifestyle. These diseases result in a condition called metabolic syndrome, which is caused by insulin resistance associated with obesity, and, rather like dominoes falling, they develop one after another. The incidence of obesity and metabolic syndrome continues to increase owing to changes in dietary habits and work environments in both developed and developing countries. Particularly in Asian countries, the problem of obesity and metabolic syndrome in people with obesity genes is a serious social issue that needs to be solved.

Studies on adipokines and batokines secreted by adipose tissue as paracrine factors have revealed the mechanisms underlying the onset of metabolic syndrome and the relationship of non-alcoholic hepatitis, cancer, and dementia with metabolic syndrome. Recently, the effects of interventions such as lifestyle modification have also been investigated.

This book deals with the latest topics related to lifestyle-related diseases and metabolic syndrome in three important ways. First, it provides an overview of the pathogenesis of metabolic syndrome and its characteristics. Second, the relationship between metabolic syndrome and hypertension, brain function, and non-alcoholic hepatitis is discussed. Finally, the therapeutic effects of herbs and interventions on lifestyle-related diseases in Japan and Africa are addressed. These chapters provide important information for the active treatment of metabolic syndrome and lifestyle-related diseases.

I would like to thank Mrs. Maja Bozicevic and the staff of IntechOpen Publishers for their invaluable support with the writing and publication of this book.

Naofumi Shiomi
Kobe College,
Nishinomiya, Japan

Chapter 1

Introductory Chapter: An Overview of Metabolic Syndrome and Its Prevention

Naofumi Shiomi

1. Introduction

Diseases, including type 2 diabetes, heart disease, hypertension, stroke, chronic renal failure, and nonalcoholic hepatitis, are caused by incorrect diet, irregular lifestyle, and environmental factors. Hence, these diseases are called "lifestyle-related diseases" in Japan. They are characterized by the onset of obesity and the concomitant development of one or more other diseases. In the group with diabetes, the risk of developing hypertension is twice and that of ischemic heart disease is approximately thrice as high. The risk of heart disease augments with an increase in the number of diverse risk factors, including obesity, diabetes, hypertension, hyperlipidemia, and heart disease, poses about 36 times higher risk when 3–4 risk factors are present simultaneously [1]. Furthermore, these diseases are known to enhance the risk of cancer, immunodeficiency, aging, and dementia, which are not directly linked to lifestyle-related diseases [2, 3]. This condition wherein diseases develop one after another, such as domino falling, triggered by obesity, is termed "metabolic syndrome (MetS)" [4].

The number of obese and MetS patients continues to rise not only in developed but also in developing countries with altering diets and environments, and it is reported that 18% of individuals over 19 years of age are obese globally [5]. According to a 2015–2016 survey in the United States, 39.8% of adults were obese, and diabetes and prediabetes rates were 9.4% and 33.9%, respectively [6]. In China, the incidence of MetS has increased by 2% in urban areas over the past decade since 1992, reaching 15.5% in 2017 [7]. According to a study by the Japanese Ministry of Health, Labor, and Welfare, one in two men and one in five women over the age of 40 years fall into MetS and its pre-groups.

In this introductory chapter of the book, I will outline (1) the mechanism of MetS and (2) recent research trends on the effective use of brown and beige adipocytes, which have gained attention as an approach for enhancing MetS reserves.

2. Mechanisms triggering MetS

White adipose tissue (WAT) predominantly contains white adipocytes that are accountable for triglyceride storage. They also serve as endocrine organs by secreting diverse hormones, including adipokines. More than 10 hormones and miRNAs, including TNF-α, PAI-1, leptin, adiponectin, resistin, apelin, and chemelin, are adipokines secreted by white adipocytes [8]. These act as paracrine and perform crosstalk with nerves and several organs to help control blood glucose and lipid levels [8, 9]. When normal body weight is maintained, the ratio of progenitor cells to white adipocytes is balanced and adipokines aid to control them with insulin. However, if excessive intake of sugar and fat pursues, progenitor cells differentiate into white adipocytes, which then enlarge and attain their fat storage limit. Under such conditions, adipokines are irregularly secreted by white adipocytes, that are unable to transmit their signals appropriately [10]. WAT hypertrophy and abnormal adipokine secretion, resulting in mild chronic inflammation and insulin resistance, cause MetS development.

Insulin resistance is defined as the inhibition of insulin-mediated signaling pathways, resulting in a hyperglycemic state. The mechanisms of insulin resistance associated with obesity are complex; however, the following are believed to be the major factors [8, 11, 12]. Due to tissue hypertrophy in obese subcutaneous fat, macrophage infiltration occurs through chemokines, including CCL2, triggering inflammation. Macrophages differentiate into M1 macrophages, which activate innate immunity and generate inflammatory mediators. Inflammatory adipokine secretion from hypertrophic WAT also augments. TNF-α and IL-6, inflammatory adipokines, activate inhibitory molecules, including SOCS and JNK, which suppress IRS and inhibit insulin signaling causing insulin resistance. Furthermore, PIP3 is degraded by phospholipid phosphatases, including PTEN, and stresses the endoplasmic reticulum, diminishing its function and inhibiting GLUT-4 migration to the plasma membrane.

Insulin resistance augments free fatty acids (FFAs) throughout the body, which strongly affect inflammation and insulin resistance [13]. The resulting ectopic deposition of FFAs in muscles and the liver results in serine phosphorylation in IRS-1, which inhibits insulin signaling. FFAs also activate the NF-κB pathway and induce inflammation. Ectopic deposition of FFA also elevates diacylglycerol levels in the liver, resulting in reduced hepatic glycogen synthesis. Conversely, white adipocytes secrete anti-inflammatory adipokines, including leptin, adiponectin, and apelin. Apelin promotes insulin sensitivity, glucose uptake, and lipolysis [14]. Recent studies have implied that obese individuals have elevated levels of leptin and apelin, thus causing resistance to these adipokines.

Persistent insulin resistance leads to abnormal glucose and lipid metabolism, resulting in high blood glucose and lipid concentrations. In the hyperglycemic state, ketone bodies are synthesized, causing type II diabetes mellitus (T2DM). Additionally, high LDL cholesterol causes adherence of oxidized lipids to blood vessels, which are phagocytosed by macrophages activated by chronic inflammation, creating plaques, thereby causing atherosclerosis. Hypertrophic WAT increases the secretion of PAI-1, an adipokine that augments blood pressure and causes hypertension. Furthermore, hyperlipidemia, triggered by enhanced FFAs levels, is the source of a variety of other diseases. Although FFAs bind to albumin and other blood proteins and are not toxic, excess FFAs impair the pancreatic mitochondria, causing dysfunction [15] and inability to secrete insulin, resulting in a more advanced form of T2DM. Chronic inflammation and disruption of the immune system cause chronic renal failure (CDK), cancer, and aging [2, 3]. Thus, MetS initiating with obesity leads to a state of insulin resistance and mild chronic inflammation, which in turn triggers consecutive development of diverse diseases.

3. Improvement of pathophysiology in metabolic syndrome

3.1 Brown and beige adipocytes

Once T2DM, atherosclerosis, or chronic renal failure develop, their reversal becomes tremendously challenging. Therefore, to prevent MetS, it is imperative to eliminate insulin resistance and chronic inflammation during the pre-metabolic syndrome stage. Here, we discuss brown and beige adipocytes, which have gained prominence as the best approach to improving metabolic syndrome.

Brown adipocytes are so named owing to their brown, muscle-like color; nevertheless, they accumulate and degrade fat rapidly. Beige adipocytes, which materialize in WAT upon cold stimulation, have an excellent ability like that of brown adipocytes but are not as brownish [16]. These adipocytes originate from different developmental lineages. Brown adipocytes are derived from Myf5+/Sca1+/Pax7+ cells in the dermis muscle layer of skeletal muscle and dermal precursors, whereas beige adipocytes are reported to emerge by trans-differentiation of WAT or differentiate from beige adipocyte precursors. Recently, it has been proposed that there may be numerous beige adipocytes depending on the WAT type [17]. Marker genes specific to brown and beige adipocytes have been found, including Cd137 and Cited1, specific for beige adipocytes, and Prdm16, Ucp1, and Pgc-1α are common markers for brown and beige adipocytes [18, 19].

Brown and beige adipocytes are heat-producing cells that generate nonshivering heat through diverse mechanisms [16, 20, 21]. In the mitochondrial inner membrane, energy, including NADH, produced by the TCA circuit is employed to pump protons outside of the membrane, creating an energy difference inside and outside the membrane for ATP synthesis. Brown and beige adipocytes have numerous mitochondria expressing uncoupling protein 1 (UCP1) in their inner membrane. On cold stimulation exposure, UCP1 opens ion channels and conjugates with anions, including long-chain fatty acids, to bring protons into the membrane. The energy lost in this process is converted to thermal energy, producing nonshivering heat. As mitochondria rush to restore the proton gradient via the TCA circuit, fatty acids are positively degraded by β-oxidation to produce acetyl CoA. In this manner, brown and beige adipocytes generate heat in response to cold stimuli, causing rapid fatty acid degradation. Although not deliberated here, mechanisms other than UCP1 that activate heat production have recently been identified and several regulators have been determined [22, 23]. This may be critical for reducing obesity, especially in the elderly and obese populations with few UCP1-positive adipocytes.

3.2 Effectiveness of brown and beige adipocytes on metabolic syndrome

It is well established that nonshivering heat produced by brown adipose tissue (BAT) is involved in thermoregulation of body temperature when animals awaken from hibernation and in humans in response to alterations in body temperature at birth. Thermogenesis by UCP1 in brown adipocytes has been observed to be closely related to obesity and T2DM [24]. For example, in mice, UCP1 does not function well in individuals prone to obesity, and UCP1 functions well in individuals that are not prone to obesity. In humans, BAT, which is abundant in newborns, drastically decreases as they grow older or develop MetS, although it plays an imperative role in maintaining health in adults. This decline is one of the reasons for the rapid rise in the incidence of MetS in adults over 40 years of age [25]. Therefore, augmenting the number of brown and beige adipocytes is expected to be an effective means of obesity and MetS [26].

Brown adipocytes not only play a role in fat metabolism through thermogenesis but have also been found to secrete cytokines, including FGF-21, follistatin, IL-6, CLCX14, or miRNA (batokines), upon thermogenic activation. Batokines work as paracrine and endocrine molecules and crosstalk with several organs [27, 28]. For example, BMP8 promotes sympathetic innervation and angiogenesis in BAT, whereas NRG4 promotes sympathetic axon elongation and secretion. FGF21 is released from BAT activated by thermogenesis and the liver, protecting against hyperlipidemia and nonalcoholic liver disease. Thermogenesis-activated BAT also secretes IL-6, which helps maintain BAT metabolic homeostasis and enhances gluconeogenesis in the liver. 12,13-dihydroxy-9Z-octadekanoic acid (12,13 diHOMO) improves cardiac function and cardiomyocyte respiration. Additionally, CLCX14 induces M2 macrophages and myostatin regulates skeletal muscle function. Thus, batokines secreted from BAT and beige adipocytes are anticipated to suppress MetS.

3.3 Signals for white adipocytes browning and inducing brown adipocytes

Activation of beige or brown adipocytes is primarily mediated by a pathway involving the β3-adrenergic receptor (β3-AR) [29]. Noradrenaline binds to β3-AR on adipocytes' surface and stimulates adenylate cyclase, which in turn activates PKA employing cAMP as a second messenger. Activated PKA phosphorylates pJMJD1A, CEBP, ATF2, and other proteins via p38 MAPK to enhance the expression of PPARγ, PGC1a, PRDM16, NFIA, and others [30]. Enhanced expression of PPARγ and PRDM16 induces browning and PGC1a augments the number of mitochondria, resulting in the induction of UCP1, CIDEAR, COX8b, CDK5, and others.

The most crucial heat-producing factor in BAT is the transcription factor PRDM16, which initiates the brown adipocyte transcriptional program when coexpressed with C/EBPβ. Experiments in mice in which PRDM16 was disrupted have demonstrated that it is vital for brown adipose tissue maintenance and WAT browning [31]. The transcription factor Zfp516 also plays a pivotal role in BAT development and cold-induced regulation. Deletion of Zfp516 in mice results in BAT development failure, while overexpression results in WAT browning and an increase in tissue oxygen consumption by more than 80% [32]. Additionally, IFR4 ablation in mice drastically decreases thermogenesis and energy consumption [33]. This indicated that IRF4 interacts with PGC1α and is involved in energy expenditure. It is noteworthy that continuous cold stimulation is essential for the differentiation of pre-brown to brown adipocytes and white to beige adipocytes. It has been reported that the modification from white to beige adipocytes is trans-differentiation, which returns to its original state once cold stimulation is stopped [34].

However, pathways have been found to activate BAT or induce beige adipocytes independent of BAT β3-AR signaling [35]. For example, adenosine A2A receptors bind to adenosine released by brown fat cells, and their activation can induce beige adipogenesis and suppress obesity [36]. Additionally, beige adipocytes differentiated from MyoD+ progenitors (glycolytic beige adipocytes) exhibit thermogenesis and energy homeostasis by adapting to cold conditions without β3-AR signaling [37]. It has also been demonstrated that UCP1 knockout mice adapt to cold environments by employing other compensatory pathways [38]. This β3-AR signaling-independent pathway will also be an imperative target for enhancing beige adipocytes in the future.

3.4 Preventive treatment of metabolic syndrome with thermogenic fat

Beige adipocytes in humans have beneficial effects in alleviating insulin resistance and weight loss [39] and treating metabolic syndrome by converting into beige adipocytes which have been attempted. The most representative approach for WAT browning is cold stimulation. Even in humans, cold exposure at 17°C every 2 h for 6 weeks augments BAT activity and reduces body fat percentage [40]. Additionally, cold stimulation for 10 days in type 2 diabetics boosted insulin sensitivity by 43% and skeletal muscle glucose uptake [41]. Thus, continuous cold stimulation is a simple and effective means to enhance BAT or beige adipocytes.

BAT activation by agonists has also been explored. Because the β3-AR of BAT acts on noradrenaline secreted by cold stimulation, β3-AR agonists also induce thermogenesis. For example, mirabegron, a β3-AR agonist, induces BAT activity and augments resting energy expenditure by up to 5.8% [42]. PPARγ receptor agonists, such as rosiglitazone, also activate SIRT1-PRDM16 and induce beige adipocyte development in mice [43]. However, β3-AR and PPARγ receptors are distributed throughout the body, and their side effects are challenging and have not yet been acknowledged for the treatment of metabolic disorders. Thus, researchers at Columbia University Medical Center are attempting to provide them specifically using a skin patch. The skin patch was equipped with several tiny needles. When applied to mice's abdomen with skin patches coated with rosiglitazone, WAT turned into beige adipocytes, resulting in a 20% fat reduction [44]. Additionally, cell therapy for direct BAT augmentation by transplantation is also being considered, as brown and beige fat cells can be produced from iPS cells and diverse other cells [45, 46].

Moreover, there is also a requirement for foods that can reduce fat and promote the activation of BAT and WAT beige [47]. Active consumption of these foods will help obtain a lean body and prevent metabolic syndrome. Because cold stimuli are received by TRP channels on the vagus nerve, compounds that stimulate TRP channels, including capsaicin, gingerol, and allyl isothiocyanate, are expected to have a cold stimuli-like effect. For example, when ingested, capsaicin or capsinoids activates the exchange nerve through its TRPV1 channel, and adrenaline is secreted [48]. When capsinoids were continuously ingested for 6 weeks, there was an increase in BAT and cold-induced heat production [40]. Additionally, EPA and DHA, or intestinal bacterial metabolites of unsaturated fatty acids, also have TRPV1 activating effects and have been reported to improve cold-induced heat production in BAT [49].

Food components with noradrenaline-like structures can stimulate β3-AR, and their continuous intake may induce brown or beige adipocytes. We reported that *Kikyo*, the constituents of *Bofutsushosan* (Chinese medicine), contain components that transdifferentiate mouse white adipocytes into beige adipocytes [50]. Another group reported that p-synephrine extracted from *Citrus unshiu Marcow* contains a component that converts to beige adipocytes [51].

It has also recently been demonstrated that sirtuins are closely involved in browning [52], SIRT3 is involved in mitochondrial function maintenance, and SIRT5 regulates UCP1. Furthermore, SIRT1 aids in the BAT gene transcription via PPARγ and activates PGC-1a [53]. Because SIRT1 is reduced by aging and age-related diseases, enhancing SIRT1 activity may prevent metabolic syndrome pathogenesis. Intravenous administration of resveratrol-bound nanoparticles targeting adipose stromal cells (ASCs) for 5 weeks significantly induced differentiation into beige adipocytes, reduction in fat mass by 40%, and enhanced glucose homeostasis and inflammation [54].

Additionally, it has been noted that chitosan, although not differentiating into beige adipocytes, acts on adipokines and has an inhibitory effect on obesity [55]. Experiments employing an animal model of diet-induced obesity indicated that chitosan oligosaccharide capsules activated the JAK2-STAT3 signaling pathway to mitigate leptin resistance, inhibit lipogenesis, and reduce lipid accumulation [56].

4. Conclusion

Obesity and MetS are becoming global diseases. The mechanisms by which MetS is caused have been elucidated. It is now comprehended that insulin resistance and mild chronic inflammation elimination are critical for MetS improvement and prevention and that augmenting brown and beige fat cells, which secrete batokines and improve insulin resistance, are vital for improving MetS. Furthermore, recent progress in research on brown and beige adipocytes has been remarkable, and existence of UCP1-independent nonshivering heat and signaling pathways that exclude β3-ARs have been demonstrated. The significance of using brown and beige adipocytes in metabolic syndrome treatment is expected to intensify in the future. We look forward to further research on brown and beige adipocytes.

Author details

Naofumi Shiomi
School of Human Sciences, Kobe College, Japan

*Address all correspondence to: n-shiomi@mail.kobe-c.ac.jp

References

[1] Nakamura T, Tsubono Y, Kameda-Takemura K, Funahashi T, Yamashita S, et al. Magnitude of sustained multiple risk factors for ischemic heart disease in Japanese employees –a case-control study. Japanese Circulation Journal. 2001;**65**:11-17

[2] Esposito K, Chiodini P, Colao A, Lenzi A, Giugliano D. Metabolic syndrome and risk of cancer: A systematic review and meta-analysis. Diabetes Care. 2012;**35**(11):2402-2411

[3] Andersen CJ, Murphy KE, Fernandez ML. Impact of obesity and metabolic syndrome on immunity. Advancers in Nutrition. 2016;**7**(1):66-75

[4] Lemieux I, Després J-P. Metabolic syndrome: Past, present and future. Nutrients. 2020;**12**(11):3501

[5] Saklayen MG. The global epidemic of the metabolic syndrome. Curr Hypertenssion Reports. 2018;**20**(2):12

[6] U.S. Dept of Health and Human Services. Center for Diseases Control and Preventation. National Diabetes Statistics Report. 2017

[7] Wang Y, Mi J, Shan X-Y, Wang QJ, Ge K-Y. Is China facing an obesity epidemic and the consequences? The trends in obesity and chronic disease in China. International Journal of Obesity. 2007;**31**(1):177-188

[8] Lee M-W, Lee M, Oh K-J. Adipose tissue-derived signatures for obesity and type 2 diabetes: Adipokines, batokines and microRNAs. Journal of Clinical Medicine. 2019;**8**(6):854

[9] Fahed G, Aoun L, Zerdan MB, Allam S, Zerdan MB, et al. Metabolic syndrome: Updates on pathophysiology and management in 2021. International Journal of Molecular Sciences. 2022;**23**(2):786

[10] Shiomi N, Maeda M, Mimura M. Compounds that inhibit triglyceride accumulation and TNFα secretion in adipocytes. Journal of Biomedical Science and Engineering. 2011;**4**(11):684-691

[11] Piya MK, McTernan PG, Kumar S. Adipokine inflammation and insulin resistance: The role of glucose, lipids and endotoxin. Journal of Endocrinology. 2013;**216**:T1-T15

[12] Kwon H, Pessin JE. Adipokines mediate inflammation and insulin resistance. Frontiers in Endocrinology. 2013;**4**:71

[13] Sears B, Perry M. The role of fatty acids in insulin resistance. Lipids in Health and Diseases. 2015;**14**:121

[14] Dray C, Knauf C, Daviaud D, Waget A, Boucher J, et al. Apelin stimulates glucose utilization in normal and obese insulin-resistant mice. Cell Metabolism. 2008;**8**(5):437-445

[15] Kim J, Wei Y, Sowers JR. Role of mitochondrial dysfunction in insulin resistance. Circulation Research. 2008;**102**(4):401-414

[16] Wang Z, Yu X, Chen Y. Recruitment of thermogenic fat: Trigger of fat burning. Frontiers in Endocrinology. 2021;**12**:696505

[17] Shao M, Wang QA, Song A, Vishvanath L, Busbuso NC, et al. Cellular origins of beige fat cells revisited. Diabetes. 2019;**68**:1874-1885

[18] Garcia RA, Roemmich JN, Claycombe KJ. Evaluation of markers of

beige adipocytes in white adipose tissue of the mouse. Nutrition & Metabolism. 2016;**13**:24

[19] Pilkington A-C, Paz HA, Wankhade UD. Beige adipose tissue identification and marker specificity—Overview. Frontiers in Endocrinology. 2021;**12**:599134

[20] Dempersmier J, Sul HS. Shades of brown: A model for thermogenic fat. Frontiers in Endocrinology. 2015;**6**:71

[21] Peng X-R, Gennemark P, O'Mahony G, Bartesaghi S. Unlock the thermogenic potential of adipose tissue: Pharmacological modulation and implications for treatment of diabetes and obesity. Frontiers in Endocrinology. 2015;**6**:174

[22] Chouchani ET, Kazak L, Spiegelman BM. New advances in adaptive thermogenesis: UCP1 and beyond. Cell Metabolism. 2019;**29**(1):27-37

[23] Ikeda K, Yamada T. UCP1 dependent and independent thermogenesis in brown and beige adipocytes. Frontiers in Endocrinology. 2020;**11**:498

[24] Brondani LA, Assmann TS, Duarte GCK, Gross JL, Canani LH, et al. The role of the uncoupling protein 1 (UCP1) on the development of obesity and type 2 diabetes mellitus. Arquivos Brasileiros de Endocrinologia & Metabologia. 2012;**56**(4):215-225

[25] Cypess AM, Lehman S, Williams G, Tal I, Rodman D, et al. Identification and importance of brown adipose tissue in adult humans. The New England Journal of Medicine. 2009;**360**(15):1509-1517

[26] Rabiee A. Beige fat maintenance; toward a sustained metabolic health. Frontiers in Endocrinology. 2020;**11**:634

[27] Villarroya J, Cereijo R, Gavaldà-Navarro A, Peyrou M, et al. New insights into the secretory functions of brown adipose tissue. Journal of Endocrinology. 2019;**243**(2):R19-R27

[28] Yang FT, Stanford KI. Batokines: Mediators of inter-tissue communication (a mini-review). Current Obesity Reports. 2022;**11**(1):1-9

[29] Cero C, Lea HJ, Zhu KY, Shamsi F, Tseng Y-H, et al. β3-adrenergic receptors regulate human brown/beige adipocyte lipolysis and thermogenesis. JCI Insight. 2021;**6**(11):e139160

[30] Cao W, Medvedev AV, Daniel KW, Collins S. Beta-adrenergic activation of p 38 MAP kinase in adipocytes: cAMP induction of the uncoupling protein 1 (UCP1) gene requires p 38 MAP kinase. Journal of Biological Chemistry. 2001;**276**(29):27077-27082

[31] Harms MJ, Ishibashi J, Wang W, Lim H-W, Goyama S, Sato T, et al. Prdm16 is required for the maintenance of brown adipocyte identity and function in adult mice. Cell Metabolism. 2014;**19**(4):593-604

[32] Dempersmier J, Sambeat A, Gulyaeva O, Paul SM, Hudak CSS, et al. Cold-inducible Zfp516 activates UCP1 transcription to promote browning of white fat and development of brown fat. Molecular Cell. 2015;**57**(2):235-246

[33] Kong X, Banks A, Liu T, Kazak L, Rao RR, Cohen P. IRF4 is a key thermogenic transcriptional partner of PGC-1α. Cell. 2014;**158**(1):69-83

[34] Rosenwald M, Perdikari A, Rülicke T, Wolfrum C. Bi-directional interconversion of brite and white adipocytes. Nature Cell Biology. 2013;**15**(6):659-667

[35] Pan R, Zhu X, Maretich P, Chen Y. Combating obesity with thermogenic fat:

Current challenges and advancements. Frontiers in Endocrinology. 2020;**11**:185

[36] Gnad T, Scheibler S, von Kügelgen I, Scheele C, Kilić A, et al. Adenosine activates brown adipose tissue and recruits beige adipocytes via A2A receptors. Nature. 2014;**516**:395-399

[37] Chen Y, Ikeda K, Yoneshiro T, Scaramozza A, Tajima K, et al. Thermal stress induces glycolytic beige fat formation via a myogenic state. Nature. 2019;**565**(7738):180-185

[38] Ukropec J, Anunciado RP, Ravussin Y, Hulver MW, Kozak LP. UCP1-independent thermogenesis in white adipose tissue of cold-acclimated Ucp1−/− mice. Journal of Biological Chemistry. 2006;**281**(42):31894-31908

[39] Huo C, Song Z, Yin J, Zhu Y, Miao X, et al. Effect of acute cold exposure on energy metabolism and activity of brown adipose tissue in humans: A systematic review and meta-analysis. Frontiers in Physiology. 2022;**13**:917084

[40] Yoneshiro T, Aita S, Matsushita M, Kayahara T, Kameya T, et al. Recruited brown adipose tissue as an antiobesity agent in humans. Journal of Clinical Investigation. 2013;**123**(8):3404-3408

[41] Chondronikola M, Volpi E, Børsheim E, Porter C, Annamalai P, et al. Brown adipose tissue improves whole-body glucose homeostasis and insulin sensitivity in humans. Diabetes. 2014;**63**(12):4089-4099

[42] Kessler H, Kahn PA, English J, Chatman K, Trauger SA, et al. Activation of human brown adipose tissue by a β3-adrenergic receptor agonist. Cell Metabolism. 2015;**21**(1):33-38

[43] Ohno H, Shinoda K, Spiegelman BM, Kajimura S. PPARγ agonists induce a white-to-brown fat conversion through stabilization of PRDM16 protein. Cell Metabolism. 2012;**15**(3):395-404

[44] Zhang Y, Liu Q, Yu J, Yu S, Wang J, et al. Locally induced adipose tissue browning by microneedle patch for obesity treatment. ACS Nano. 2017;**11**(9):9223-9230

[45] Brown AC. Brown adipocytes from induced pluripotent stem cells—How far have we come? Annals. New York Academy of Sciences. 2020;**1463**(1):9-22

[46] Lu K-Y, Dass KTP, Lin S-Z, Harn H-J, Liu S-P. The application of stem cell therapy and brown adipose tissue transplantation in metabolic disorders. Cytotherapy. 2020;**22**(10):521-528

[47] Kawarasaki S, Takahashi H, Kawada T, Goto T. Thermogenesis via the food factors-induced activation of brown adipose tissue functions (Japanese). Trace Nutrients Research. 2018;**35**:98-104

[48] Yang F, Zheng J. Understand spiciness: Mechanism of TRPV1 channel activation by capsaicin. Protein & Cell. 2017;**8**(3):169-177

[49] Kim M, Goto T, Yu R, Uchida K, Tominaga M, et al. Fish oil intake induces UCP1 upregulation in brown and white adipose tissue via the sympathetic nervous system. Scientific Reports. 2016;**5**:18013

[50] Shiomi N, Ito M, Watanabe K. Characteristics of beige adipocytes induced from white adipocytes by *Kikyo* extract. Journal of Biomedical Science and Engineering. 2016;**9**(7):342-353

[51] Takagi M, Kimura K, Nakashima K, Hirai T, Inoue M. Induction of beige adipocytes by naturally occurring β3-adrenoceptor agonist p-synephrine.

European Journal of Pharmacology. 2018;**836**:67-74

[52] Favero G, Krajčíková K, Rezzani R. Browning of adipose tissue and sirtuin involvement. In: Leszek Szablewski edtor. In Adipose Tissue. Rejeca. INTECH 2018. pp. 51-72

[53] Wang GX, Meyer JG, Cai W, Softic S, Mengyao ME, et al. Regulation of UCP1 and mitochondrial metabolism in brown adipose tissue by reversible succinylation. Molecular Cell. 2019;**74**(4):844-857.e7

[54] Zu Y, Zhao L, Hao L, Mechref Y, Zabet-Moghaddam Y, et al. Browning white adipose tissue using adipose stromal cell-targeted resveratrol-loaded nanoparticles for combating obesity. Journal of Controlled Release. 2021;**333**:339-351

[55] Walsh AM, Sweeney T, Bahar B, O'Doherty JV. Multi-functional roles of chitosan as a potential protective agent against obesity. PLoS One. 2013;**8**(1):e53828

[56] Pan H, Fu C, Huang L, Jiang Y, Deng X, et al. Anti-obesity effect of chitosan oligosaccharide capsules (COSCs) in obese rats by ameliorating leptin resistance and adipogenesis. Marine Drugs. 2018;**16**(6):198

Chapter 2

Immune System and Inflammation in Hypertension

Mohammed Ibrahim Sadik

Abstract

Hypertension is a widely prevalent and a major modifiable risk factor for cardiovascular diseases. Despite the available long list of anti-hypertension drugs and lifestyle modification strategies for blood pressure control, a large number of hypertensive patients fail to achieve adequate blood pressure control even when prescribed a combination of drugs from three or more classes. Thus, identifying and targeting of further mechanisms that underlie hypertension is decisive in alleviating burden of this disorder. In recent decades research have shown that perturbed immune system and inflammation contribute to hypertension. Experimental studies on animal models have shown that immune cells such as dendritic cells, macrophages, and lymphocytes contribute for the development and/or sustaining of hypertension. In hypertension, inflammatory immune cells that infiltrated the kidney cause retention of sodium, renal fibrosis, glomerular injury, and chronic kidney disease, all of them contribute for elevated blood pressure. Similarly, immune cells and inflammatory cytokines are involved in blood vessels structural and functional changes associated with hypertension. Perturbed immune system and chronic low-grade systemic inflammation enhance SNS activity and this contributes to elevated blood pressure by its effect on blood vessels tone, on the kidneys, and on immune system.

Keywords: hypertension, immune system, inflammation

1. Introduction

Hypertension is defined as office or clinic systolic blood pressure (SBP) values >140 mmHg and/or diastolic blood pressure (DBP) values >90 mmHg in adult population [1, 2]. It is one of the major modifiable risk factors for cardiovascular diseases (CVDs) [3]. Hypertension is the main risk factor for cardiovascular diseases, especially for coronary heart disease, heart failure, arrhythmia, stroke, peripheral vascular disease, and also for chronic kidney disease and dementia [4]. Globally, in the year 2017, high systolic blood pressure was the leading risk factor of all-cause deaths, accounting for 10.4 million deaths and 218 million disability-adjusted life-years (DALYs), followed by smoking, high fasting plasma glucose (FPG), high body-mass index (BMI), and short gestation for birth weight. Astonishingly, from 1990 to 2017, high SBP was consistently responsible for the largest number of all-cause deaths, followed by smoking and high FPG respectively [5]. In 2010, 31.1% (1.39 billion people) of the world's adults had hypertension [6]. The number of adults with hypertension in 2025 was predicted to be a total of 1.56 billion [7].

Currently, hypertension treatment drugs such as adrenoceptor antagonists (propranolol and prazosin), ACE inhibitors (perindopril), angiotensin receptor blockers (irbesartan), mineralocorticoid antagonists (spironolactone), diuretics (thiazides and amiloride), and vasodilators (nitrates, calcium channel blockers, and hydralazine) are being used to control blood pressure in hypertensive patients [8]. Despite, the presence of a plethora of antihypertensive drugs and lifestyle modification strategies for blood pressure control a large number of hypertensive patients remained undiagnosed or untreated or did not control their blood pressure to target level in spite of being treated [6]. The proportion of hypertensive population that got treatment (55.6% in high-income countries (HIC), 29.0% in low and middle-income countries (LMIC)) and that got their blood pressure controlled (28.4% in HIC, 10.3% in LMIC) is astonishingly low [9]. Moreover, up to 40% of patients with hypertension fail to achieve adequate blood pressure control, even when prescribed a combination of drugs from three or more classes [10]. These observations highlight lack of efficacy of the current hypertension prevention and control strategies and also indicate that in some patients at least, additional drivers of hypertension must exist, and new targets need to be identified and targeted for the treatment of hypertension.

Hypertension is associated with chronic low-grade systemic inflammation [11]. It is hypothesized that perturbation in immune system and chronic low-grade systemic inflammation is one of the contributors in development and/or sustaining of hypertension. Accordingly, this book chapter composed existing evidence to show the contribution of perturbation in immune system and chronic low-grade systemic inflammation to the development and/or sustaining of hypertension.

2. Immune system and inflammation in hypertension

2.1 Inflammation and immunity basics

Inflammation is an immune system response to noxious stimuli entered or occurred in a tissue that includes pathogens, damaged cells, toxic compounds, or irradiation; and inflammation acts to remove the noxious agent and to initiate healing process. At tissue level, inflammation is characterized by swelling, redness, heat, pain, and loss of tissue function, which are considered five cardinal signs of inflammation, and these signs result due to local immune, vascular, and inflammatory cells response to infection or injury [12]. In addition to infection and tissue injury, inflammation can be initiated due to disruption of cellular and tissue homeostasis. It has been shown that cells with disrupted homeostasis that undergoes senescence release inflammatory mediators known as the senescence associated secretory phenotypes (SASP). While excessive cell stress such as ER, mitochondrial or osmotic stress that cannot be handled by effector mechanisms within homeostatic regime activates NLRP3 inflammasome [13]. Recently, researchers are mentioning inflammation as a spectrum of a system (organism, tissues, cells) state; homeostatic state, stress response state, and inflammatory state. Indeed, both stress response and inflammation are engaged to eliminate the stressor (i.e., the source of perturbation), to promote adaptations to the stressor, and ultimately to return the system to the homeostatic state [14]. Deviations of regulated variables within a normal range are corrected by the homeostatic circuit (including stress responses) while extreme deviations of regulated variables beyond the homeostatic range trigger the inflammatory response [13]. At the same time, it is important to notice that even though inflammation brings homeostatic state at the end, inflammation and inflammatory mediators are both antagonistic to and dominant over homeostatic signals [14].

Thus, inflammation can be induced by extreme deviations in regulated variables of cellular and tissue homeostasis or by agents that cause disruption of tissue homeostasis, including pathogens, toxins, and xenobiotics [14]. The inflammation process is coordinated by a large range of mediators that form complex regulatory networks. Inflammatory pathway is composed of inflammation inducers, inflammation sensors, inflammation mediators, and inflammatory effectors [15].

Inflammation is a component of the broader and wider immune system. The immune system is composed of a complex network of specialized cells where each type has precise roles. The immune system is an interactive network of lymphoid organs, cells, humoral factors, and cytokines [16]. The immune system has two lines of defense, innate immunity, and adaptive immunity. Innate immunity is nonspecific defense mechanism which is used by the host immediately or within hours of encountering an antigen. It comprises four types of defensive barriers: anatomic (skin and mucous membrane), physiologic (temperature, low pH, and chemical mediators), endocytic and phagocytic, and inflammatory [17]. Innate immunity relies upon a repertoire of germline-encoded receptors, the pattern recognition receptors (PRRs) that recognize the pathogen-associated molecular patterns (PAMPs) to detect microbial structures and the damage-associated molecular patterns (DAMPs) to detect immunological danger (molecules released during the cell lysis and tissue damage) [18]. Innate immunity rapidly recruits immune cells to sites of infection and induces inflammation through the production of cytokines (tumor necrosis factor (TNF), interleukin 1 (IL-1) and interleukin 6 (IL-6)) and chemokines [17]. Moreover, innate immunity is considered as an ingenious doorbell that awakens the adaptive immune response through antigen-presenting cells (APCs) such as dendritic cells (DCs) that present antigens to the lymphocytes (with the optimal T cell receptor (TCR) specificity and affinity) and also costimulatory signals, which guarantee full proliferation and differentiation of the lymphocytes [19]. Adaptive immunity consists of two broad sets of antigen-responsive cells, the B and T lymphocytes. B lymphocytes are the precursors of antibody-producing cells, plasma cells. Antibodies are capable of recognizing three-dimensional structures and thus can interact with and lead to the neutralization of pathogens in extracellular fluid. By contrast, the T cell antigen recognition system recognizes a complex consisting of an antigen-derived peptide bound into a specialized groove in class I and class II major histocompatibility complex (MHC) molecules of APCs [20]. CD8+ T cells can interact with peptides (9–11 amino acids in length) on almost any cell expressing MHC class I while the TCRs of CD4+ T cells engage peptides bearing MHC class II. The activated T cells can play direct roles in elimination of pathogens by killing infected target cells, they can function by providing cognate (involving direct cellular contact) or cytokine signals to enhance both B- and T-cell responses, as well as causing activation of mononuclear phagocytes, and also T cells regulate immune responses, limiting tissue damage incurred by means of autoreactive or overly inflammatory immune responses [21]. In adaptive immunity, long-lived memory cells (memory lymphocytes) ensure that a second encounter with the same invader is dealt with swiftly and effectively because of the greater number (for the given antigen), extended lifespan, more rapid response rate, superior proliferation capacity, and wider access to tissues of the memory lymphocytes [19].

2.2 Inflammatory cytokines in hypertension

Inflammation plays a vital role in preserving physiological homeostasis of an organism, in protection against invading agents such as bacteria and virus, and in healing processes of damaged tissue. On the other hand exaggerated inflammation or chronic inflammation can cause tissue damage, and contributes for the development and/or persistence of many diseases [22]. Acute inflammatory response can be initiated during times of infection or in response to physical, chemical, or metabolic noxious stimuli through interaction between pattern recognition receptors expressed on innate immune cells and PAMPs or DAMPs. On the other hand, chronic low-grade systemic inflammation is typically triggered in the absence of an acute infectious insult [23].

Chronic low grade systemic inflammation is a low-grade, systemic, unresolved, and smoldering chronic inflammation clearly indicated by a 2- to 4-fold increase in serum levels of inflammatory mediators, including interleukin-6 (IL-6) and acute phase proteins, for example, C-reactive protein (CRP); even though there is no numerical cut off values for elevated inflammatory mediators to define chronic low grade systemic inflammation at the present time [24]. In chronic low grade systemic inflammation, besides CRP and IL-6, a large number of cellular (total leukocytes, granulocytes, and activated monocytes) and pro- and anti-inflammatory mediators including IL-1, IL-8, IL-13, IL-18, interferon-α and interferon-β, tumor necrosis factor, CC chemokine ligands, adhesion molecules, and acute-phase reactants (serum amyloid A, and fibrinogen) are involved or are produced as a result of the inflammatory processes. Chronic low grade systemic inflammation is associated with many chronic disease conditions including CVDs, neurodegenertion and Alzheimer's disease, insulin resistance and type 2 diabetes mellitus, tumorigenesis and cancer, osteoporosis, anemia, chronic kidney disease, depression, sarcopenia, and disability [25].

Whereas hypertension has predominantly been ascribed to perturbations of the vasculature, kidney, and central nervous system, researches have shown that the immune system also contributes to this disease. Inflammatory cells that accumulate in the kidneys and vasculature of humans and experimental animal models with hypertension likely contribute not only for pathogenesis of hypertension but also contribute to end-organ damage [26].

An association between hypertension and inflammation has been clearly demonstrated while it is not clear whether inflammation is predominantly a cause or an effect of hypertension [11]. Many studies indicated that an inflammatory marker CRP level increases as blood pressure level increases. A prospective follow up study done on 15, 215 women found that, in cross-sectional analyses of baseline data of the study, increasing categories of blood pressure were significant predictors of CRP levels; meaning linear increase in levels of CRP was seen as levels of systolic blood pressure or diastolic blood pressure increases [27]. Another case-control study done among 904 participants, 39–50 years old, found a continuous, independent association between serum CRP and elevated blood pressure. The study also reported that, after adjustment for sex, obesity, race, serum insulin level and family history of coronary heart disease, odds ratios for hypertension increased progressively across CRP quintiles; participants in the highest CRP quintile were 2.35 times more likely to have hypertension than those in the lowest quintile [28]. Similarly, a case-control study done on 1529 subjects (767 hypertensive and 762 non-hypertensive) aged from 30 to 84 years, reported that the means for BP and CRP in cases (hypertensive subjects) were significantly higher than that in controls (non-hypertensive subjects) [29]. A study carried out on 335 non-hypertensive study participants, with mean arterial blood pressure of 135/85 mmHg and age of 65 years at base line, indicated that the 2-year risk for new-onset hypertension was 18% greater for 1 mg/l increment of CRP after adjustment for low-density lipoprotein cholesterol and BMI [30]. A prospective cohort study done on 20,525 female USA health professionals aged 45 years or above found that the adjusted relative risk (RR) of developing hypertension is 1.5 for the group with the highest level of CRP at base line compared with the group of the lowest CRP at the base line. From their cohort study, the study group concluded that CRP levels are associated with future development of hypertension [31].

Similar to association trend observed between CRP and blood pressure, higher level of other pro-inflammatory cytokines were reported among hypertensive population or individuals with higher blood pressure (BP) levels compared with non-hypertensive population or individuals with lower BP levels. A study done on 79 hypertensive and 117 non-hypertensive study subjects showed that plasma Il-6 and TNF-α were significantly higher (two to four times higher) in hypertensive subjects compared to non-hypertensive subjects [32]. Similarly, another study that assessed association of blood pressure level with plasma concentrations of soluble intercellular adhesion molecule-1 (sICAM-1) and interleukin-6 (IL-6) among 508 apparently healthy men, found increasing levels of SBP, pulse pressure (PP), and mean arterial pressure (MAP) were significantly associated with increased levels of sICAM-1 while all blood pressure parameters (SBP, DBP, PP, MAP) were significantly associated with increasing levels of IL-6 [33]. Two independent studies that compared the serum and the peripheral blood mononuclear cells (PBMCs) IL-1β levels among hypertensive and non-hypertensive groups found significantly higher level of IL-1β among hypertensive groups [34, 35].

Experimental studies on animals also confirmed association between hypertension and inflammation. An experimental study that compared blood pressure levels among angiotensin II (Ang II) infused mice (wild type mice versus IL-6 deficient mice (IL6−/−) found that in wild-type mice systolic blood pressure began to increase by day 3, increased significantly by day 7, reached a peak by day 10, and continuously maintained high blood pressure through the end of 2-week Ang II infusion while genetic deletion of IL-6 in mice led to a significant reduction of Ang II-induced hypertension [36]. Another experimental study showed that RNA interference knockdown of IL-6 in Sprague-Dawley rats abolished the cold-induced upregulation of IL-6 in kidney and aorta, and also significantly attenuated cold-induced elevation of systolic blood pressure [37].

An experimental study that compared effect of Ang II to infusion into wild types (WT) mice and TNF-α knockout (KO) (TNF-α−/−) mice found that Ang II infusion for 14 days significantly increased mean arterial pressure in WT mice from (115 ± 1 to 151 ± 3 mmHg) but not in TNF-α−/− mice (113±2 to 123±3 mm Hg). The study also showed that, when TNF-α−/− mice are given replacement therapy with human recombinant TNF-α, Ang II administration caused an increase in mean arterial pressure (109 ± 1 to 153 ± 3 mm Hg) [38]. Another experimental study done on mice, which compared blood pressure level among angiotensin II infused WT mice and type 1 interleukin-1 receptor (IL-1R1)-deficient (KO) mice showed that during chronic Ang II infusion, the IL-1R1 KO animals were partially protected from hypertension compared to the WT controls (165±6 versus 180±3 mmHg). The study also reported administering an IL-1R1 antagonist (anakinra) or vehicle to WT mice for 3 days prior to and during chronic Ang II infusion resulted in IL-1R1 blockade with anakinra significantly attenuated the level of blood pressure elevation during chronic Ang II infusion (154 ± 4 versus 167 ± 3 mmHg). Both isoforms of IL-1 (IL-1α and IL-1β) bind and signal via the IL-1R1 [39].

An experimental study that investigated effect of a proinflammatory cytokine interleukin 17 (IL17) reported that initial hypertensive response was similar for wild type mice (C57BL/6J mice) and interleukin 17 deficient mice (IL17−/− mice) however hypertension was not sustained in IL17−/− mice, reaching levels 30 mmHg lower than in wild type mice by 4 weeks of angiotensin II infusion. Moreover, blood vessels from IL17−/− mice displayed preserved vascular function, decreased superoxide production, and reduced aortic T cell infiltration in response to angiotensin II infusion which is indicative for importance of IL17 for the maintenance of angiotensin II-induced hypertension and vascular dysfunction [40].

2.3 Innate and adaptive immunity cells in hypertension

In addition to above mentioned human and animal studies that showed association between inflammatory cytokines and hypertension, many studies implicated that both innate and adaptive immunity cells play roles in hypertension pathophysiology.

Variability, diversity, and joining (V(D)J) recombination is the specialized DNA rearrangement used by cells of the immune system to assemble immunoglobulin and T-cell receptor genes from the preexisting gene segments. The RAG1 and RAG2 proteins are the only lymphoid-specific factors needed for V(D)J recombination that generate diverse B-lymphocytes antibodies and T-cell receptors [41]. An experimental study on mice showed that in mice with genetic deletion of the recombinase-activating gene (RAG-1−/−) mice, mice that lack both T and B lymphocytes, hypertension caused by chronic low-dose angiotensin II infusion was markedly blunted. Similar to response for angiotensin II infusion, in the experimental study, the increase in blood pressure was also blunted in RAG-1-/- mice in desoxycorticosterone acetate (DOCA) – salt hypertension model, indicating that lymphocytes likely play a role in different types of hypertension. Besides, in the RAG-1−/− mice study, adoptive transfer of B cells into RAG-1−/− mice had little effect on the increase in blood pressure while adoptive transfer of T cells restored the hypertension response to angiotensin II infusion. This study indicated that the T lymphocyte plays a critical role in the development of hypertension [42].

A study done on mice showed that infusion of angiotensin II for 14 days into wild type (WT), CD4−/−, and CD8−/− mice resulted in blunted blood pressure increase in CD8−/− mice while WT and CD4−/− mice exhibited increased blood pressure in response to angiotensin II. The study also reported that an increase in blood pressure in response to deoxycorticosterone acetate (DOCA)-salt challenge was significantly reduced in CD8−/− mice compared to either CD4−/− or WT mice, similar to angiotensin II-induced hypertension response [43]. It is known that mice lacking CD4 (CD4−/− mice) also lack regulatory T cells (Tregs) which may predispose to aggravated hypertension in CD4−/− mice in the above mentioned experimental study [43].

Osteopetrotic (Op/Op) mice have no colony-stimulating factor 1 gene and thus they lack colony-stimulating factor l (CSF-1), and are functionally deficient in macrophages [44]. In an experimental study done on adult Op/Op, heterozygous (Op/+), and wild type (+/+) mice, infusion of Ang II for 14-days resulted in significantly increased blood pressure in wild type (+/+) and heterozygous (Op/+) mice while blood pressure in Op/Op remained unaffected from base line level [45]. Similarly, in a study where Op/Op, heterozygous (Op/+), and wild type (+/+) mice given deoxycorticosterone acetate (DOCA)-salt for 14 days, systolic blood pressure (mmHg) was significantly increased (146 +/− 2 and 138 +/− 1; P < 0.001 vs. basal 115 +/− 3 and 115 +/− 3) in wild-type (+/+) and heterozygous (Op/+) mice respectively, but not in Op/Op mice (130 +/− 1 vs. basal 125 +/− 3) [46].

In an experimental study which selectively ablated lysozyme M-positive (LysM+) myelomonocytic cells by low-dose diphtheria toxin in mice with inducible expression of the diphtheria toxin receptor (LysM iDTR), thus the experimental group of mice have reduced number of monocytes in the circulation of the mice without affecting number neutrophils, showed that attenuated Ang II-induced blood pressure increase among experimental group compared to control group [47].

Activation of T cells requires two signals; the first involves interaction of the T cell receptor with an antigenic peptide presented in the context of major histocompatibility complex on antigen-presenting cells (APCs) while the second, referred to as costimulation, involves the simultaneous interaction of receptors in proximity to the TCR with ligands on the APC. Among several potential costimulatory interactions, the binding of T cell CD28 and cytotoxic T-lymphocyte-associated protein 4 (CTLA-4) (CD152) with B7 ligands CD80 and CD86 on APCs is important, particularly for activation of naïve T cells [48]. A study done on mice showed that blockade of B7-dependent costimulation of T-cells with CTLA4-Igl reduced both angiotensin II- and DOCA-salt induced hypertension. Moreover, in mice lacking B7 ligands (B7−/− mice), due to genetic deletion of both CD80 and CD86, angiotensin II caused minimal blood pressure elevation and vascular inflammation, and these effects were restored by transplant with wild-type bone marrow. This study indicated that stimulation of T-cells by dendritic cells is important in both angiotensin II- and DOCA-salt induced hypertension [49].

A study was done on mice that are genetically deficient of B cells, B-cell–activating factor receptor-deficient (BAFF-R−/−) mice, showed that while Ang II infusion caused a rapid rise in SBP from 117 ± 3 mmHg at baseline to a maximum level of 165 ± 5 mmHg by day 21 in wild type mice, the pressor response to Ang II was attenuated in BAFF-R−/− mice with SBP reaching a maximum of only 149 ± 4 mm Hg at day 21 and remaining at this level until day 28 from the base BP level 112 ± 3 mm Hg. Moreover, the study showed that the introduction of B cells into BAFF-R−/− mice were sufficient to fully recapitulate the pressor response to Ang II to levels observed in wild-type mice. This study demonstrated that B cells are crucial for the development of Ang II-induced hypertension [50]. Mutations in the BAFF-R are associated with B-cell lymphopenia and antibody deficiency.

In an experimental study done on Ang II-induced hypertension mice model, mice injected with CD4+CD25+ regulatory T cells (CD4+CD25+ Tregs) and infused with hypertension doses of Ang II (400 ng/kg/min) for 2 weeks showed significantly lower increment in blood pressure compared with mice that infused only hypertension doses of Ang II [51]. Similarly, another study on mice reported that mice injected CD4+CD25+ regulatory T cells (CD4+CD25+ Tregs) three times, at two-week intervals and then infused with Ang II for 14 days showed blunted increase of SBP compared with control group (group that did not receive regulatory T cells) [52]. In another experimental study that compared blood pressure change among mice received aldosterone infusion and 1% saline in drinking water, mice that infused with aldosterone and received Treg cells adoptive transfer did not show significant increase in both systolic and diastolic blood pressure when compared with control group mice (control mice were similarly injected intravenously with vehicle and received tap drinking water); while mice group that was infused with aldosterone and given 1% saline in drinking water without receiving Treg cells showed significant increase in both systolic and diastolic blood pressure compared to control group [53]. On contrary to the above mentioned study results one experimental study on mice reported that mice that received Treg cells and infused with Ang II showed similar incitement in blood pressure with group of mice that infused Ang II without receiving transfer of Treg cells [54]. The different results of the latter study may be due to differences in experiment procedures as all former studies performed Treg cells transfer few weeks before infusion of Ang II or aldosterone while the latter study performed Treg cells transfer and Ang II infusion simultaneously.

Thus, the existing body of knowledge clearly confirmed existence of association between immune system activation and hypertension while ascertaining the cause effect relationship between inflammation and hypertension needs further study.

2.4 Mechanisms that underlie association between immune system perturbation and chronic inflammation, and hypertension

An individual's blood pressure is largely determined by the functions of three key organs, namely the heart which pumps blood through the circulatory system, the blood vessels which regulate blood flow through the organs and the whole body, and the kidneys which regulate sodium and water excretion and hence blood volume. The maintenance of physiological blood pressure levels involves coordinated control and regulation from neurohormonal system which includes the renin-angiotensin-aldosterone system (RAAS), the natriuretic peptides and the endothelium, the sympathetic nervous system (SNS) and the immune system on functions of the heart, blood vessels and the kidneys. Perturbation in function of organs or systems that are involved in BP control can directly or indirectly lead to increase in blood pressure that ultimately ends up in the development of hypertension, and over time results in target organ damage such as, left ventricular hypertrophy and chronic kidney disease (CKD) and CVD outcomes [55].

Existing observational and experimental studies highlight that in some hypertensive patients at least, additional drivers of hypertension must exist than the already known mechanisms involved in pathophysiology of hypertension, and new targets must be defined [10]. Inflammation and immune system perturbation are likely contributors in the development and sustaining of hypertension. The current overarching hypothesis about inflammation and immune system involvement in pathophysiology of hypertension is that immune cells accumulation in blood vessels (in particular, in the perivascular fat), kidneys, heart, and brain promote a chronic inflammatory response that disrupts the blood pressure-regulating functions of these organs, leading to hypertension [56]. Accordingly, inflammation and immune system activation cause derangement in kidneys, arteries, brain, and heart functions that consequently promote hypertension and end-organ damage [57].

In support of the above mentioned hypothesis, current studies indicated that known stimuli that raise blood pressure (such as high-salt diet, Ang II, and DOCA-salt) directly and indirectly activate immune system cells. Elevated blood pressure can stress tissue cells to the level that DAMPs released by tissues. Moreover, hypertensive stimuli can directly activate immune cells and also cause formation of neoantigens in the tissues. As a result of released DAMPs, neoantigens, and direct immune cells activation by hypertension stimuli, activated immune cells are formed, target organs infiltrated by activated immune cells, and diverse inflammatory cytokines are released by the activated immune cells. Eventually, the affected target organs, mainly the kidney, blood vessels, and sympathetic nervous system function are perturbed and this leads to further elevated blood pressure level and finally to hypertension. Immune cells such as monocytes, macrophages, and dendritic cells (DCs) release pro-hypertensive cytokines that promote the BP elevation via actions in the vasculature (augmenting vascular dysfunction), kidney (increasing sodium retention), and stimulating sympathetic nervous system outflow [58].

Many studies implicated that in the kidney, inflammatory cells and their products contribute to blood pressure elevation at least in part by increasing renal sodium transport [59].

Genetic deletion of IL-6 in mice results in blunted hypertension in response to angiotensin II infusion [60]. Treating cortical collecting duct cells culture with IL-6 (100 ng/ml) for 12 h caused increased expression and activity of the epithelial sodium channel (ENaC) [61]. Mutations in ENaC that increase sodium reabsorption lead to the development of high blood pressure in Liddle's syndrome (a rare inherited form of hypertension) while mutations that inactivate ENaC have also been identified in humans, and these mutations lead to low blood pressure [62]. Taken together, these studies suggest that IL-6 enhances renal tubule sodium reabsorption and elevates BP at least in part through up regulation of renal tubule ENaC.

IL-1 is a pro-inflammatory cytokine that plays a central role in both acute and chronic inflammation, acting as a primary inducer of the innate immune response. Studies indicated that type 1 IL-1 receptor (IL-1R1) stimulation by IL-1 potentiates blood pressure elevation by suppressing nitric oxide (NO)-dependent sodium excretion in the kidney. Nitric oxide is a potent driver of sodium excretion in the kidney that acts via cyclic guanosine monophosphate (cGMP) and phosphodiesterase two to limit Na-K-2Cl cotransporter (NKCC2) activity in the medullary thick ascending limb. Thus, by relieving NO inhibitory effect on NKCC2, IL-1 enhances reabsorption of electrolytes by medullary thick ascending limb and enhances retention of sodium and water by kidney [39].

Interferon gamma (IFN-γ) is a proinflammatory cytokine produced by innate and adaptive immune cells, and T cell production of IFN-γ is increased in Ang II-induced hypertension and mice deficient in IFN-γ have a blunted blood pressure response to Ang II infusion. Experimental studies indicate that IFN-γ positively regulates sodium hydrogen exchanger 3 (NHE3) in the proximal tubule, NKCC2 in medullary thick ascending limb, and NCC in the distal tubule. Whether IFN-γ directly modulates these sodium transporters or acts through downstream mediators is unknown [62].

Interleukin 17A (IL-17A) is a pro-inflammatory cytokine produced predominantly by CD4+ T helper 17 (Th17) cells as well as gamma delta T cells. An experimental study that investigated effect of a proinflammatory cytokine interleukin 17 (IL17) reported that initial hypertensive response was similar for wild type mice (C57BL/6J mice) and interleukin 17 deficient mice (IL17−/− mice) however hypertension was not sustained in IL17−/− mice in Ang II hypertension model [40]. Mice model experimental studies and cell culture model studies showed that interleukin 17A up regulates NHE3 (in proximal segment), NCC and ENaC (in distal segment) of renal tubules. Moreover, studies implicated that interleukin 17A regulates renal sodium transporters through a serum and glucocorticoid regulated kinase 1 (SGK1) dependent pathway [63]. Serum and glucocorticoid regulated kinase1 is an important mediator of salt and water retention in the kidney through inhibition of neural precursor cell expressed developmentally down-regulated 4-2 (Nedd4-2) mediated ubiquitination and degradation of NHE3, NCC, and ENaC in the renal tubule, thereby enhancing the expression of these transporters on the cell surface [64].

Besides its effect on electrolyte and water homeostasis regulation function of kidney, sustained inflammation results in renal fibrosis, oxidative stress, glomerular injury, and chronic kidney disease [59].

Blood vessels are other organs that are affected by activated immune system and chronic low grade inflammation associated with hypertension. Elevated blood pressure has an impact on the vasculature as a consequence of both the mechanical effects of blood pressure and shear stress [65]. Inflammation can impair blood vessels in two ways. Inflammation can cause functional arterial stiffening by impairing the functional relaxation capability of arteries. The other mechanism is structural remodeling of arteries due to hypertension-associated inflammation [66]. Likewise, many experimental studies confirmed involvement of immune cells and inflammatory cytokines in vascular dysfunction associated with experimental hypertension.

An experimental study done on mice showed that Ang II infusion in mice increased immune cell content (T cells, macrophages, and dendritic cells) in perivascular adipose tissue and adventitia [67].

Endothelial cell culture study showed that inflammatory marker, C-reactive protein (CRP), caused a marked down regulation of endothelial nitric oxide synthase (eNOS) mRNA and protein expression [68]. Similarly, TNF-α mediated inhibition of eNOS expression was observed in endothelial cell culture [69]. Acute treatment of endothelial cells with IL-17 caused a significant increase in phosphorylation of the inhibitory eNOS residue threonine 495 (eNOS Thr495) [70]. All these studies indicate that inflammation decreases bioavailability of endothelial NO and thus impairs vascular smooth muscle relaxation and subsequent vasodilatations.

Moreover, involvement of immune cells and inflammatory cytokines in hypertensive vascular remodeling is implicated by many studies. Reduced vascular remodeling showed in Ang II or DOCA- salt induced hypertension in osteopetrosis (Op/Op) mice [10]. In RAG1−/− mice (mice deficient in T and B lymphocytes) reduced aortic and small artery remodeling observed in response to Ang II-induced hypertension [41]. Similarly, interleukin 17A deficient (IL-17a−/−) mice are protected against aortic collagen deposition and aortic stiffening in response to chronic angiotensin II infusion [71]. These studies implicated that immune cells and inflammatory cytokines play roles in vascular fibrosis, remodeling of small and large vessels, and vascular rarefaction in hypertension. Nonetheless, this remains to be further investigated.

Other important organ both in development of hypertension and as an end-organ target of hypertension is the brain. Regulation of short-term blood pressure level by sympathetic nervous system (SNS) is well established. SNS stimulation is associated with constriction of blood vessels, increased cardiac output, and augmented sodium and fluid retention by the kidneys [72]. Moreover, SNS serves as an integrative interface between the brain and the immune system.

Mounting evidence implicate that many forms of essential hypertension are initiated and maintained by an elevated sympathetic tone [73]. The elevated sympathetic activity can be initiated by several factors including humoral factors such as angiotensin II and by environmental factors such as stress and high salt intake. In view of sympathetic nervous system substantial innervation to both primary (thymus, bone marrow) and secondary (spleen, lymph nodes, Peyer's patches) lymphoid tissues, and the central nervous system (CNS) powerful influences on the immune system and vice versa, it is reasonable to suppose that CNS enhance immune responses that lead to hypertension [74]. Pro-inflammatory cytokines (such as TNF-α, IL-1β) produced in the periphery can signal to the brain, passing through the BBB at points of increased permeability in the circumventricular organs (CVOs) and/or through disrupted blood brain barrier (BBB), and results in increased sympathetic outflow [75].

Observations such as increased splenic sympathetic nerve discharge (SND) and consequent increase in splenic cytokine gene expression (IL-1β, IL-6, IL-2, and IL-16) due to central Ang II administration (the effect which was abrogated by splenic sympathetic denervation), and others led to the hypothesis that central stimuli such as angiotensin II cause modest elevations of blood pressure, which leads to activation of immune system. Subsequently, the activated immune system leads to severe hypertension [76]. This hypothesis proposed a mechanism that occurs in a two-phase feed forward fashion. The initial phase brings a modest elevation in blood pressure (i.e. pre-hypertension), giving rise to an inflammatory response, possibly by generating "neoantigens" that activate innate and adaptive immune system. In the second phase, the activated immune system generates cytokines and other inflammatory mediators which work in concert with the direct effects of hypertensive stimuli (such as angiotensin II, catecholamines, and salt) to cause vascular and renal dysfunction, promote vasoconstriction, vascular remodeling, a shift in the pressure natriuresis curve and sodium retention, and ultimately causes sustained hypertension [74].

3. Conclusion

Hypertension is a widely prevalent public health problem of world adult population. It is a major risk factor of cardiovascular diseases, chronic kidney disease, and dementia. Despite the availability of a plethora of hypertensive drugs, up to 40% of patients with hypertension fail to achieve adequate blood pressure control, even when prescribed a combination of drugs from three or more classes. This indicates lack of efficacy of existing hypertension treatment strategies and existence of additional drivers of hypertension that must be identified and may be targeted.

One of the proposed pathophysiologic mechanisms that contribute for elevated BP and target organ damage among hypertensive patients is activation of the immune system and chronic low grade systemic inflammation.

In kidneys, inflammatory cells and their products contribute to blood pressure elevation by increasing renal sodium retention and by causing renal fibrosis, oxidative stress, and glomerular injury. IL-1, IL-6, IFN-γ, and IL-17 are among pro-inflammatory cytokines that enhance sodium retention by renal tubules.

Activated immune cells and pro-inflammatory cytokines may contribute to functional arterial stiffening and structural remodeling of arteries that consequently cause elevated blood pressure in hypertension. C-reactive protein, TNF-α, and IL-17 may hamper synthesis of or inhibit nitric oxide (NO) synthase. Inflammatory cells that infiltrate blood vessels such as macrophages and lymphocytes and their pro-inflammatory products may also contribute for vascular remodeling.

Perturbed immune system and chronic low grade systemic inflammation also enhance SNS activity which in turn contributes to elevated blood pressure by its effect on blood vessels tone (vasoconstriction), on the kidneys (sodium and water retention, RAAS activation) and on immune system (activation of immune system and enhanced production pro-inflammatory cytokines).

Thus, unraveling the detail pathophysiological mechanisms by which activated immune system and inflammation contribute to hypertension paves a way to identify target, and to design and develop therapeutic intervention for hypertension.

Even though currently there is no anti-inflammatory drug to treat hypertension, anti-inflammatory agents that target specific inflammatory pathway (without compromising general immune system of an individual) are possible future hypertension treatment drugs.

Conflict of interest

Author does not have any conflict of interest whatsoever with regard to content or opinions expressed above.

Author details

Mohammed Ibrahim Sadik
Jimma University, Jimma, Oromia, Ethiopia

*Address all correspondence to: mohaisadik@yahoo.com

References

[1] Williams B, Mancia G, Spiering W, Agabiti RE, Azizi M, Burnier M, et al. 2018 ESC/ESH Guidelines for the management of arterial hypertension: The Task Force for the management of arterial hypertension of the European Society of Cardiology (ESC) and the European Society of Hypertension (ESH). European Heart Journal. 2018;**39**(33):3021-3104

[2] Unger T, Borghi C, Charchar F, Khan NA, Poulter NR, Prabhakaran D, et al. 2020 international society of hypertension global hypertension practice guidelines. Hypertension. 2020;**75**(6):1334-1357

[3] Fuchs FD, Whelton PK. High blood pressure and cardiovascular disease. Hypertension. 2020;**75**(2):285-292

[4] paho.org/en [internet]. [Cited on July 1, 2021]. Available from: https://www.paho.org/en/events/world-hypertension-day-17-may-2021

[5] Stanaway JD, Afshin A, Gakidou E, Lim SS, Abate D, Abate KH, et al. Global, regional, and national comparative risk assessment of 84 behavioural, environmental and occupational, and metabolic risks or clusters of risks for 195 countries and territories, 1990-2017: A systematic analysis for the Global Burden of Disease Study. The Lancet. 2017;**392**(10159):1923-1994

[6] Mills KT, Bundy JD, Kelly TN, Reed JE, Kearney PM, Reynolds K, et al. Global disparities of hypertension prevalence and control: A systematic analysis of population-based studies from 90 countries. Circulation. 2016;**134**(6):441-450

[7] Kearney PM, Whelton M, Reynolds K, Muntner P, Whelton PK, He J. Global burden of hypertension: Analysis of worldwide data. The Lancet. 2005;**365**(9455):217-223

[8] Whelton PK, Carey RM, Aronow WS, Casey DE, Collins KJ, Dennison HC, et al. 2017 ACC/AHA/AAPA/ABC/ACPM/AGS/APhA/ASH/ASPC/NMA/PCNA guideline for the prevention, detection, evaluation, and management of high blood pressure in adults: A report of the American College of Cardiology/American Heart Association Task Force on Clinical Practice Guidelines. Journal of the American College of Cardiology. 2018;**71**(19):e127-e248

[9] Geldsetzer P, Manne GJ, Marcus ME, Ebert C, Zhumadilov Z, Wesseh CS, et al. The state of hypertension care in 44 low-income and middle-income countries: A cross-sectional study of nationally representative individual-level data from 1.1 million adults. Lancet. 2019;**394**:652-662

[10] Wenzel UO, Ehmke H, Bode M. Immune mechanisms in arterial hypertension. Recent advances. Cell and Tissue Research. 2021;**385**(2):393-404

[11] Dinh QN, Drummond GR, Sobey CG, Chrissobolis S. Roles of inflammation, oxidative stress, and vascular dysfunction in hypertension. BioMed Research International. 2014;**2014**:1-11

[12] Chen L, Deng H, Cui H, Fang J, Zuo Z, Deng J, et al. Inflammatory responses and inflammation-associated diseases in organs. Oncotarget. 2018;**9**(6):7204-7218

[13] Meizlish ML, Franklin RA, Zhou X, Medzhitov R. Tissue homeostasis and inflammation. Annual Review of Immunology. 2021;**39**:557-581

[14] Chovatiya R, Medzhitov R. Stress, inflammation, and defense of homeostasis. Molecular Cell. 2014;**54**(2):281-288

[15] Medzhitov R. Origin and physiological roles of inflammation. Nature. 2008;**454**(7203):428-435

[16] Parkin J, Cohen B. An overview of the immune system. The Lancet. 2001;**357**(9270):1777-1789

[17] Marshall JS, Warrington R, Watson W, Kim HL. An introduction to immunology and immunopathology. Allergy, Asthma & Clinical Immunology. 2018;**14**(2):1-10

[18] Turvey SE, Broide DH. Innate immunity. The Journal of Allergy and Clinical Immunology. 2010;**125**(2):S24-S32

[19] Yatim KM, Lakkis FG. A brief journey through the immune system. Clinical Journal of the American Society of Nephrology. 2015;**10**(7):1274-1281

[20] Paul WE. Bridging innate and adaptive immunity. Cell. 2011;**147**(6):1212-1215

[21] Bonilla FA, Oettgen HC. Adaptive immunity. The Journal of Allergy and Clinical Immunology. 2010;**125**(2): S33-S40

[22] Rönnbäck C, Hansson E. The importance and control of low-grade inflammation due to damage of cellular barrier systems that may lead to systemic inflammation. Frontiers in Neurology. 2019;**10**:533

[23] Furman D, Campisi J, Verdin E, Carrera BP, Targ S, Franceschi C, et al. Chronic inflammation in the etiology of disease across the life span. Nature Medicine. 2019;**25**(12):1822-1832

[24] Tkacova R. Systemic inflammation in chronic obstructive pulmonary disease: may adipose tissue play a role? Review of the literature and future perspectives. Mediators of Inflammation. 2010;**2010**:1-11

[25] Chen Y, Liu S, Leng SX. Chronic low-grade inflammatory phenotype (CLIP) and senescent immune dysregulation. Clinical Therapeutics. 2019;**41**(3):400-409

[26] Trott DW, Harrison DG. The immune system in hypertension. Advances in Physiology Education. 2014;**38**(1):20-24

[27] Blake GJ, Rifai N, Buring JE, Ridker PM. Blood pressure, C-reactive protein, and risk of future cardiovascular events. Circulation. 2003;**108**(24):2993-2999

[28] Bautista LE, Atwood JE, O'Malley PG, Taylor AJ. Association between C-reactive protein and hypertension in healthy middle-aged men and women. Coronary Artery Disease. 2004;**15**(6):331-336

[29] Xu T, Ju Z, Tong W, Hu W, Liu Y, Zhao L, et al. Relationship of C-reactive protein with hypertension and interactions between increased C-reactive protein and other risk factors on hypertension in Mongolian people. Chinese Circulation Journal. 2008;**72**(8):1324-1328

[30] Dauphinot V, Roche F, Kossovsky MP, Schott AM, Pichot V, Gaspoz JM, et al. C-reactive protein implications in new-onset hypertension in a healthy population initially aged 65 years: the Proof study. Journal of Hypertension. 2009;**27**(4):736-743

[31] Sesso HD, Buring JE, Rifai N, Blake GJ, Gaziano JM, Ridker PM. C-reactive protein and the risk of

developing hypertension. The Journal of the American Medical Association. 2003;**290**(22):2945-2951

[32] Bautista LE, Vera LM, Arenas IA, Gamarra G. Independent association between inflammatory markers (C-reactive protein, interleukin-6, and TNF-α) and essential hypertension. Journal of Human Hypertension. 2005;**19**(2):149-154

[33] Chae CU, Lee RT, Rifai N, Ridker PM. Blood pressure and inflammation in apparently healthy men. Hypertension. 2001;**38**(3):399-403

[34] Dalekos GN, Elisaf M, Bairaktari E, Tsolas O, Siamopoulos KC. Increased serum levels of interleukin-1β in the systemic circulation of patients with essential hypertension: Additional risk factor for atherogenesis in hypertensive patients? Journal of Laboratory and Clinical Medicine. 1997;**129**(3):300-308

[35] Zhao S, Li Q, Liu L, Xu Z, Xiao J. Simvastatin reduces interleukin-1β secretion by peripheral blood mononuclear cells in patients with essential hypertension. Clinica Chimica Acta. 2004;**344**(1-2):195-200

[36] Zhang W, Wang W, Yu H, Zhang Y, Dai Y, Ning C, et al. Interleukin 6 underlies angiotensin II–induced hypertension and chronic renal damage. Hypertension. 2012;**59**(1):136-144

[37] Crosswhite P, Sun Z. Ribonucleic acid interference knockdown of interleukin 6 attenuates cold-induced hypertension. Hypertension. 2010;**55**(6):1484-1491

[38] Sriramula S, Haque M, Majid DS, Francis J. Involvement of tumor necrosis factor-α in angiotensin II–mediated effects on salt appetite, hypertension, and cardiac hypertrophy. Hypertension. 2008;**51**(5):1345-1351

[39] Zhang J, Rudemiller NP, Patel MB, Karlovich NS, Wu M, McDonough AA, et al. Interleukin-1 augments salt retention in angiotensin II-induced hypertension via nitric oxide-dependent regulation of the NKCC2 sodium co-transporter. Cell Metabolism. 2016;**23**(2):360-368

[40] Madhur MS, Lob HE, McCann LA, Iwakura Y, Blinder Y, Guzik TJ, et al. Interleukin 17 promotes angiotensin II–induced hypertension and vascular dysfunction. Hypertension. 2010;**55**(2):500-507

[41] Gellert M. V (D) J recombination: RAG proteins, repair factors, and regulation. Annual Review of Biochemistry. 2002;**71**(1):101-132

[42] Guzik TJ, Hoch NE, Brown KA, McCann LA, Rahman A, Dikalov S, et al. Role of the T cell in the genesis of angiotensin II–induced hypertension and vascular dysfunction. Journal of Experimental Medicine. 2007;**204**(10):2449-2460

[43] Trott DW, Thabet SR, Kirabo A, Saleh MA, Itani H, Norlander AE, et al. Oligoclonal CD8+ T cells play a critical role in the development of hypertension. Hypertension. 2014;**64**(5):1108-1115

[44] Begg SK, Radley JM, Pollard JW, Chisholm OT, Stanley ER, Bertoncello I. Delayed hematopoietic development in osteopetrotic (op/op) mice. Journal of Experimental Medicine. 1993;**177**(1):237-242

[45] De Ciuceis C, Amiri F, Brassard P, Endemann DH, Touyz RM, Schiffrin EL. Reduced vascular remodeling, endothelial dysfunction, and oxidative stress in resistance arteries of angiotensin II–infused macrophage colony-stimulating factor–deficient mice: Evidence for a

role in inflammation in angiotensin-induced vascular injury. Arteriosclerosis, Thrombosis, and Vascular Biology. 2005;**25**(10):2106-2113

[46] Ko EA, Amiri F, Pandey NR, Javeshghani D, Leibovitz E, Touyz RM, et al. Resistance artery remodeling in deoxycorticosterone acetate-salt hypertension is dependent on vascular inflammation: Evidence from m-CSF-deficient mice. American Journal of Physiology-Heart and Circulatory Physiology. 2007;**292**(4):H1789-H1795

[47] Wenzel P, Knorr M, Kossmann S, Stratmann J, Hausding M, Schuhmacher S, et al. Lysozyme M–positive monocytes mediate angiotensin II–induced arterial hypertension and vascular dysfunction. Circulation. 2011;**124**(12):1370-1381

[48] Najafian N, Sayegh MH. CTLA4-Ig: a novel immunosuppressive agent. Expert Opinion on Investigational Drugs. 2000;**9**(9):2147-2157

[49] Vinh A, Chen W, Blinder Y, Weiss D, Taylor WR, Goronzy JJ, et al. Inhibition and genetic ablation of the B7/CD28 T-cell costimulation axis prevents experimental hypertension. Circulation. 2010;**122**(24):2529-2537

[50] Chan CT, Sobey CG, Lieu M, Ferens D, Kett MM, Diep H, et al. Obligatory role for B cells in the development of angiotensin II–dependent hypertension. Hypertension. 2015;**66**(5):1023-1033

[51] Matrougui K, Kassan M, Choi S, Nair D, Gonzalez VR, Chentoufi AA, et al. Natural regulatory T cells control coronary arteriolar endothelial dysfunction in hypertensive mice. The American Journal of Pathology. 2011;**178**(1):434-441

[52] Barhoumi T, Kasal DA, Li MW, Shbat L, Laurant P, Neves MF, et al. T Regulatory lymphocytes prevent angiotensin ii–induced hypertension and vascular injury. Hypertension. 2011;**57**(3):469-476

[53] Kasal DA, Barhoumi T, Li MW, Yamamoto N, Zdanovich E, Rehman A, et al. T regulatory lymphocytes prevent aldosterone-induced vascular injury. Hypertension. 2012;**59**(2):324-330

[54] Kvakan H, Kleinewietfeld M, Qadri F, Park JK, Fischer R, Schwarz I, et al. Regulatory T cells ameliorate angiotensin II–induced cardiac damage. Circulation. 2009;**119**(22):2904-2912

[55] Suzanne O, Maria CA, George LB, Dan RB, Renata C, Anna FD, et al. Hypertension. Nature Reviews Disease Primers. 2018;**14**(4):18014

[56] Drummond GR, Vinh A, Guzik TJ, Sobey CG. Immune mechanisms of hypertension. Nature Reviews Immunology. 2019;**19**(8):517-532

[57] Norlander AE, Madhur MS, Harrison DG. The immunology of hypertension. Journal of Experimental Medicine. 2018;**215**(1):21-33

[58] Lu X, Crowley SD. Inflammation in salt-sensitive hypertension and renal damage. Current Hypertension Reports. 2018;**20**(12):1-8

[59] Norlander AE, Madhur MS. Inflammatory cytokines regulate renal sodium transporters: How, where, and why? American Journal of Physiology-Renal Physiology. 2017;**313**(2):F141-F144

[60] Lee DL, Sturgis LC, Labazi H, Osborne JJ, Fleming C, Pollock JS, et al. Angiotensin II hypertension is attenuated in interleukin-6 knockout mice. American Journal of Physiology-Heart

and Circulatory Physiology. 2006;**290**(3):H935-H940

[61] Li K, Guo D, Zhu H, Hering SK, Hamm LL, Ouyang J, et al. Interleukin-6 stimulates epithelial sodium channels in mouse cortical collecting duct cells. American Journal of Physiology-Regulatory, Integrative and Comparative Physiology. 2010;**299**(2):R590-R595

[62] Baker EH. Ion channels and the control of blood pressure. British Journal of Clinical Pharmacology. 2000;**49**(3):185-198

[63] Norlander AE, Saleh MA, Kamat NV, Ko B, Gnecco J, Zhu L, et al. Interleukin-17A regulates renal sodium transporters and renal injury in angiotensin II–induced hypertension. Hypertension. 2016;**68**(1):167-174

[64] Lang F, Stournaras C, Alesutan I. Regulation of transport across cell membranes by the serum-and glucocorticoid-inducible kinase SGK1. Molecular Membrane Biology. 2014;**31**(1):29-36

[65] Savoia C, Schiffrin EL. Hypertensive vascular disease. In: Schiffrin EL, Touyz RM, editors. Hypertension. London, UK: Future Medicine Ltd; 2013. pp. 132-150

[66] Zanoli L, Briet M, Empana JP, Cunha PG, Mäki PK, Protogerou AD, et al. Vascular consequences of inflammation: A position statement from the ESH Working Group on Vascular Structure and Function and the ARTERY Society. Journal of Hypertension. 2020;**38**(9):1682-1698

[67] Mikolajczyk TP, Nosalski R, Szczepaniak P, Budzyn K, Osmenda G, Skiba D, et al. Role of chemokine RANTES in the regulation of perivascular inflammation, T-cell accumulation, and vascular dysfunction in hypertension. FASEB Journal. 2016;**30**(5):1987-1999

[68] Verma S, Wang CH, Li SH, Dumont AS, Fedak PW, Badiwala MV, et al. A self-fulfilling prophecy: C-reactive protein attenuates nitric oxide production and inhibits angiogenesis. Circulation. 2002;**106**(8):913-919

[69] Yan G, You B, Chen SP, Liao JK, Sun J. Tumor necrosis factor-α downregulates endothelial nitric oxide synthase mRNA stability via translation elongation factor 1-α 1. Circulation Research. 2008;**103**(6):591-597

[70] Nguyen H, Chiasson VL, Chatterjee P, Kopriva SE, Young KJ, Mitchell BM. Interleukin-17 causes Rho-kinase-mediated endothelial dysfunction and hypertension. Cardiovascular Research. 2013;**97**(4):696-704

[71] Wu J, Thabet SR, Kirabo A, Trott DW, Saleh MA, Xiao L, et al. Inflammation and mechanical stretch promote aortic stiffening in hypertension through activation of p38 mitogen-activated protein kinase. Circulation Research. 2014;**114**(4):616-625

[72] Fisher JP, Paton JF. The sympathetic nervous system and blood pressure in humans: Implications for hypertension. Journal of Human Hypertension. 2012;**26**(8):463-475

[73] Guyenet PG. The sympathetic control of blood pressure. Nature Reviews Neuroscience. 2006;**7**(5):335-346

[74] Marvar PJ, Lob H, Vinh A, Zarreen F, Harrison DG. The central nervous system and inflammation in hypertension. Current Opinion in Pharmacology. 2011;**11**(2):156-161

[75] Winklewski PJ, Radkowski M, Wszedybyl WM, Demkow U. Brain

inflammation and hypertension: The chicken or the egg? Journal of Neuroinflammation. 2015;**12**(1):1-7

[76] Ganta CK, Lu N, Helwig BG, Blecha F, Ganta RR, Zheng L, et al. Central angiotensin II-enhanced splenic cytokine gene expression is mediated by the sympathetic nervous system. American Journal of Physiology-Heart and Circulatory Physiology. 2005;**289**(4):H1683-H1691

Chapter 3

Dietary Patterns for the Treatment of Arterial Hypertension in Patients with Metabolic Syndrome

António Gerson Bastos Francisco, Isaura da Conceição Almeida Lopes, Amílcar Bernardo Tomé da Silva and Henrique Cotchi Simbo Muela

Abstract

Metabolic syndrome (MetS) refers to the commonly occurring disorder comprising central obesity, systemic hypertension (HTN), insulin resistance, atherogenic dyslipidemia specifically hypertriglyceridemia, and reduced levels of high-density lipoprotein cholesterol (HDL). The prevalence of MetS worldwide ranges from 20% to 25% in the adult population and 0% to 19.2% in children, but it can reach almost 80% in type 2 diabetes patients. Increased blood pressure (BP) is considered an important component of MetS. More than 85% of those with MetS, even in the absence of diabetes mellitus (DM), have elevated BP or HTN. Dietary patterns, such as Mediterranean-style, dietary approaches to stop hypertension (DASH), low-carbohydrate, and low-fat diets, can improve insulin resistance and MetS. Dietary patterns high in fruit and vegetable content were generally found to be associated with a lower prevalence of MetS. Evidence reinforces that DASH, Nordic diet, and Mediterranean diet (MD) significantly lowered systolic BP and diastolic BP by 4.26 and 2.38 mm Hg, respectively. Therefore, we aim to review the available evidence on the effect of dietary patterns on the treatment of HTN in patients with MetS.

Keywords: dietary pattern, diet, hypertension, treatment, control, MetS

1. Introduction

Metabolic syndrome (MetS) is a growing public health problem worldwide, which is associated with an increased risk of cardiovascular morbidity and mortality [1–4]. Although many classifications have been proposed for the diagnosis of MetS, the one proposed by the International Diabetes Federation (IDF), which defines MetS as the combination of clinical and metabolic factors, including insulin resistance, hyperglycemia, hypertension (HTN), dyslipidemia, and abdominal obesity, is the most used.

Many researchers consider MetS as a transitional stage prior to organ dysfunction and death from many associated diseases, such as diabetes mellitus (DM) and cardiovascular disease (CVD) [1]. Dietary pattern is an essential element associated with MetS components, such as HTN, dyslipidemia, obesity, diabetes, and consequently CVD [3, 4]. Several studies have reported that an unhealthy diet is associated with higher CVD risk factors, and a healthy dietary pattern is associated with lower risk [2, 4]. Dietary patterns with processed food and red meat have been linked to metabolic factors and CVD, whereas a Mediterranean diet (MD) is beneficial to metabolic risk factors [3, 4].

HTN is the main MetS risk factor that leads to increased cardiovascular morbidity and mortality and is additionally an important risk factor for the development of chronic kidney disease in the presence of obesity, MetS, and microalbuminuria [1]. The association between high BP and MetS is strongly linked to the causative pathway of obesity. Blood pressure (BP) control in persons with MetS may prevent a significant number of coronary heart disease events. The primary step of treatment is lifestyle intervention with reduced caloric intake and increased physical activity. In hypertensive patients, the presence of MetS is associated with higher noncontrolled HTN levels [1], while the optimal antihypertensive treatment has been debated for years.

The relationship between dietary patterns and MetS risk factors is well-established, as indicated by recent meta-analyses [5, 6], and evidence considerably varied across populations. While a "healthy" dietary pattern (a diet rich in high vegetables, fruits, and fish consumption) was inversely associated with MetS [7], a "western" dietary pattern—high consumption of processed food and red meat, refined grains, alcohol and fried foods, increased the risk of MetS [8].

Globally, it was estimated that a quarter of the world's adult population had high BP in 2002, and the prevalence is estimated to increase to 29% by 2025 [9]. The prevalence of obesity and other MetS components in many low and middle-income countries has dramatically increased in the past decade [10]. These include the rising prevalence of HTN and obesity which are the main risk factors for cardiovascular diseases such as heart diseases and stroke worldwide [11].

Several studies have tried to bring more insight into the dietary determinants of MetS [12, 13]. Some of their limitations include a relatively small sample size of the studies, [13, 14] lack of diversity of the populations [15], limitations in the generalizability of the findings [15], and a single-nutrient approach [12, 13], whereas diet by definition is complex. Dietary pattern analysis has emerged as an attractive alternative approach for examining the effect of overall diet reflecting the eating behaviors of the population in the real world, as a result of more recognition of limitations inherent to the single nutrient approach [16]. In the assessment of dietary patterns, using instruments such as principal component analysis (PCA) allows to identify groups of nutrients through the creation of secondary variables representative of nutrients that are often consumed together. These quantitative secondary variables representative of different dietary patterns can be used in subsequent analysis to explore the relationship between specific dietary patterns and MetS. However, the latter approach is also limited by its inability to detect the predictive power of significant single nutrients, which may not be grouped with the other more complex dietary patterns. With this study, we aim to review the effect of dietary patterns on HTN treatment in patients with MetS.

2. Prevalence of metabolic syndrome in the general population and hypertensive patients

MetS is a booming global problem, with an increasing prevalence in many developing countries mainly in the urban populations [17, 18]. It is estimated that approximately one-fourth of the adult European population has MetS, with a similar prevalence in Latin America [19]. Likewise, MetS is considered an emerging epidemic in developing East Asian countries, including Korea, Japan, and China. In this region, the prevalence of MetS is estimated to range from 8% to 13% in men and from 2% to 18% in women, according to the definitions used.

The prevalence of the MetS is increasing in parallel with the growing epidemic of obesity. Almost two-thirds of the population in 2008 were overweight or obese in the United States with more than 25% of the population meeting the diagnostic criteria for MetS [19]. Comparative survey data from the late 1990s and early 2000s (1999–2000 data) showed that the age-adjusted prevalence of MetS among US adults aged 20 years and older increased from 27% (1988–1994 data) to 32% [20]. The 2011–2014 National Health and Nutrition Examination Survey (NHANES) data showed a crude estimated prevalence of 36.5% for adult obesity (32.3% in adults aged 20–39 years, 40.2% in those aged 40–59 years, and 37.0% in those aged ≥60 years) [21]. These data also showed that the overall prevalence of obesity in women was 38.3% and 34.3% in men. Among children and adolescents aged 2–19 years old, there was a prevalence of obesity of around 17% in the same period (8.9% from 2 to 5 years old, 17.5% from 6 to 11 years old, and 20.5% from 12 to 19 years old) [21].

Luckily, since this peaked in the early 2000s (2001–2002 data), the overall prevalence of MetS in the United States has dropped, mainly because of a decrease in the prevalence of hypertriglyceridemia and HTN—and despite the increase in the prevalence of hyperglycemia and obesity/waist circumference prevalence [22]. Data from the 2009–2010 NHANES reported that the age-adjusted prevalence of MetS had decreased to approximately 24% in men and 22% in women [23].

MetS is becoming more common even in African populations where the burden of disease was mainly from infectious diseases [24, 25]. Among a group of hypertensive Nigerians, the prevalence of MetS, according to three different definitions, was reported to be 34.3% according to the ATP III definition for MetS, 35% according to the WHO definition, and 42.9% according to the IDF definition [24, 26]. These rates were generally similar to those reported in the Turkish study that included nondiabetic adults, where the prevalence rates were as follows: 38% according to the NCEP-ATP III definition, 42% according to the American College of Endocrinology (ACE) and IDF definition, 20% according to the EGIR definition, and 19% according to the WHO definition [26] These values are comparable with those reported in Canada, where one-third of adult patients between 40 and 60 years old met the criteria for the MetS [27].

In the United States, African Americans have a higher prevalence of MetS, particularly African American women, and this has been attributed to the higher prevalence of obesity, HTN, and diabetes in this subgroup [28]. However, it was in Mexican Americans that the highest prevalence of age-adjusted MetS was found, where approximately one-third (31.9%) of them met the diagnostic criteria for MetS, compared with 27% of the general population, according to data from a study in 1988–1994 [20].

The prevalence of the MetS is similar in both men (24%) and women (22%), after adjusting for age [23]. However, several considerations have to be taken into account in women with MetS, including pregnancy, use of oral contraceptives, and polycystic ovarian syndrome [29].

The prevalence of MetS increases as the population ages, with about 40% of elderly people over 60 years old meeting the criteria for MetS [20]. However, MetS can no longer be considered a disease for adult populations only. Evidence published in the last decades indicates that both MetS and DM are increasingly prevalent in the pediatric population, and this growth has been recorded in parallel with the increase in the prevalence of obesity [30].

The presence of high BP is one of the required criteria for the diagnosis of MetS, while evidence also suggests that people with MetS are more likely to have HTN [31]. Results from the Pressioni Arteriose Monitorate E Loro Associazioni (PAMELA) study showed that high BP was the most frequent component of MetS in the patients who participated in the study, and it was found in more than 80%. Furthermore, participants with MetS were more prone to have higher home, office, and ambulatory BP values compared to those without MetS. All-cause mortality was also more prevalent in the population with MetS [32].

Conversely, a significant number of patients with HTN simultaneously fulfill the criteria for the diagnosis of MetS. Results from the Progetto Ipertensione Umbria Monitoraggio Ambulatoriale (PIUMA) study reported that about 34% of the hypertensive patients included also had MetS, and these patients were reported to have more cardiovascular events than those without MetS [33]. In a population-based study with more than 60,000 participants (39,998 men and 20,756 women) with no personal history of cardiovascular disease, who had a health check-up at the IPC Center (Paris, France) between 1999 and 2002, the prevalence of MetS increased proportionally with the increase in BP values [34]. After a 10-year follow-up of participants in the PAMELA study without MetS, the masked and sustained HTN based on ambulatory measurements were all associated with a higher incidence of new-onset MetS [35].

Studies conducted in the African region have consistently reported an increased prevalence of MetS in hypertensive patients despite the still high burden of infectious diseases. Tadewos et al. [36], in their study carried out in Southern Ethiopia reported that the prevalence of MetS was 48.7% and the rate was comparable with the study report from Nigeria, which was 45.6% [20]. This prevalence was even higher among hypertensive women, 54.1% which was similar to the prevalence reported in Nigeria, 54% [37].

3. Vascular pathophysiology of hypertension in metabolic syndrome

The pathogenic mechanisms linked to MetS are complex and remain to be fully explained. It is still debated whether the individual components of MetS represent different pathologies or expressions of the same pathogenic mechanism. Abdominal obesity is the main trigger for most of the mechanisms involved in MetS, thus highlighting the importance of a high caloric intake as the main causative factor [38]. Of all the proposed mechanisms, insulin resistance, neurohormonal activation, and chronic inflammation seem to be the leading players in the initiation, progression, and transition from MetS to cardiovascular disease.

The excitatory effects of insulin on the sympathetic nervous system seem to be centrally mediated, as they are observed only during systemic insulin infusion, but not during local infusion [39]. In addition, high insulin levels increase sodium reabsorption [40] favoring the extracellular fluid volume expansion, which may increase the risk of arterial HTN [41]. Furthermore, obesity leads to impaired renal-pressure natriuresis and causes sodium retention. Obese individuals require higher BP to preserve sodium balance, indicating impaired renal-pressure natriuresis [42].

The increase of epidemiological studies linking insulin resistance and hyperinsulinemia has sustained the idea of the so-called insulin hypothesis of HTN. There is no doubt that epidemiological studies have linked insulin resistance to HTN [38, 43]. The insulin hypothesis of HTN states that the compensatory hyperinsulinemia that happens with insulin resistance increases sodium reabsorption and sympathetic activity, which combine to raise the BP. Much evidence supporting this hypothesis comes from different studies. First, the correlation between insulin resistance and high blood pressure [44], is emphasized by the fact that even lean persons with essential HTN may have insulin resistance and hyperinsulinemia. Some authors go a step further by claiming that essential HTN is by itself a state of insulin resistance [45]. Second, insulin has multiple actions on the sympathetic nervous system, kidneys, and vasculature bed that may lead to HTN. Third, many drugs that improve insulin resistance and decrease hyperinsulinemia are reported to have antihypertensive effects. For instance, Landin et al. reported in their study that hypertensive men increased insulin sensitivity and significantly decreased arterial pressure after oral administration of metformin to insulin resistant [46]. Another notable example is the known BP lowering effects of the insulin sensitizers glitazones [47]. Finally, it is known that insulin sensitivity is increased by some antihypertensives drugs, such as angiotensin II-converting enzyme inhibitors [48] or angiotensin II receptor antagonists [49]. Despite the large body of evidence supporting the insulin hypothesis of HTN, there is also important evidence against it. For example, the study by Hall and collaborators failed to find a correlation between insulin and HTN in a well-controlled model in dogs [50].

In addition to insulin, leptin is also associated with the relationship between obesity and increased sympathetic activity. Apart from its effect on appetite and metabolism, leptin has actions on the hypothalamus to increase BP through the sympathetic nervous system activation mechanism [51]. Higher circulating levels of leptin are reported to explain the increase in the renal sympathetic tone seen in obese patients [52]. Evidence indicates that the leptin-induced increases in renal sympathetic activity and BP are mediated by the ventromedial and dorsomedial hypothalamus [53].

The finding that leptin or obesity receptor is expressed by the endothelium [54], transformed endothelial cells, just like those of the hypothalamus, into a target for this hormone. The presence of leptin receptors in the vascular endothelium and not only in the central nervous system is important because it allows finding a link between leptin and impaired vascular function in obese individuals [55]. Leptin is a nitric oxide-dependent vasodilator but also increases peripheral vascular resistance and sympathetic nerve activity [56]. The concentration of leptin in plasma is correlated with adiposity, and hyperleptinemia is indeed considered an independent risk factor for cardiovascular disease [57].

Finally, in visceral obese patients, high circulating levels of free fatty acids may induce the activation of the sympathetic nervous system. The increases in the release of free fatty acids into the portal vein from lipolysis in visceral fat depots may explain the association between visceral obesity and increased sympathetic nerve outflow in these patients [58].

The discovery of the role of adipose tissue as an endocrine organ has gained important implications in the understanding of the pathophysiological relationship between excess body fat and HTN [58]. Nearly all systemic arteries are surrounded by a layer of perivascular adipose tissue (PVAT). In myographic studies, PVAT is routinely removed, and this custom is based on the assumption that PVAT can prevent the diffusion of vasoactive substances. This is perhaps the reason that despite the great presence of PVAT, very little is known about its function in vascular physiology.

4. Dietary pattern, nutrients intake, and metabolic syndrome

Diet, as an important part of lifestyle, has been shown to be significantly associated with different components of MetS [59]. Dietary patterns high in fruit and vegetable content are generally associated with a lower prevalence of MetS. Otherwise, dietary patterns with high meat intake are frequently associated with increased components of MetS, particularly impaired glucose tolerance [5, 59].

The extent to which the consumption of an individual component in the diet is associated with MetS is an issue that still needs to be clarified; however, some studies suggest that dietary quality appears to play a more important role.

The Isle of Ely study [60] was a population-based study of type 2 diabetes and metabolic disorders in men and women from the Isle of Ely in the United Kingdom. Researchers used this cohort to investigate the relationship between dietary patterns and components of MetS in 802 adults aged 40–65 years [60]. The study used PCA to isolate four dietary patterns from food frequency questionnaire data, and related these patterns to components of the MetS. Four diet patterns were derived through the calculation of factor loadings for the variance of frequency for each food most commonly consumed: (a) Diet 1 (fruit, salad, fish (not fried), other vegetables, poultry, green vegetables, pasta/rice, and ice cream), (b) Diet 2 (cakes, sweets, root, vegetables, biscuits, puddings/pies, pulses, green vegetables, chocolate, and cheese), (c) Diet 3 (chocolate, sweets, crisps, cheese, soda, and fruit), and (d) Diet 4 (eggs, fried food, sausages, cheese, fried fish, nuts, and other vegetables).

According to the results from this study, both diets 1 and 2 were inversely associated with each component of the MetS. After adjustment for age, those with a higher score for diet 1 had a lower risk for increased waist–hip ratio (WHR), impaired glucose tolerance, increased plasma triglycerides and type 2 diabetes, and lower risk for decreased high-density lipoprotein cholesterol (HDL)–cholesterol. Otherwise, diets 3 and 4 had no significant associations with different components of MetS. In general, the Isle of Ely Study suggests that eating patterns characterized by high intake of fruit, vegetables, and whole cereals, and low intake of fried foods seemed to be linked to a lower risk of MetS components. Bread and milk were not specifically mentioned as part of a dietary pattern [60].

The Malmö Diet and Cancer Study [61] examined data from a sample (N = 1122) of men and women aged between 45 and 68 years that were analyzed for associations between dietary patterns and MetS components [61]. The dietary patterns that were used in this study differed significantly from that of the Isle of Ely study, possibly due to cultural habits and differences in diet, but also due to study design. Six dietary patterns were identified based on the highest proportion of energy intake from food groups, unlike the previous Isle of Ely study, which was based on the frequency of consumption. Differences in dietary patterns are to be expected, as food groups that contribute a high proportion of energy to the diet would not need to be consumed frequently to be rated high in this analysis (e.g., a high-energy chocolate bar compared to a low-energy piece of broccoli).

The relationship between dietary patterns and components of MetS differed significantly between men and women. Many foods and drinks patterns, with moderate energy intake from cheese and fat meat, were associated with an increased risk of hyperglycemia and central obesity in men. Men who scored highly for this dietary pattern had an odds ratio (OR) of 1.64 (95% CI 1.24–2.17) for hyperglycemia, while women showed no significant association. The "Fiber bread" dietary pattern with high energy intake from fiber-rich bread and fat meat was associated with a decreased risk of central obesity in men (OR 0.61, 95% CI 0.42–0.89). For women, the "White bread" dietary pattern was associated with an increased risk of hyperinsulinemia (OR 1.39, 95% CI 1.02–1.89), while the "Milk fat" dietary pattern was associated with a reduced risk of hyperinsulinemia (OR 0.58, 95% CI 0.40–0.84).

In the CARDIA study, Pereira et al. [62] investigated associations between food groups and MetS as part of the multicenter CARDIA project in the United States. The researchers of the CARDIA study did not identify dietary patterns instead, they evaluated food groups and nutrients and their influence on the onset of new cases of MetS and its components. A strong inverse association was found between consumption of dairy foods and the risk of MetS, particularly in overweight subjects. After controlling for demographic features, non-dietary lifestyle factors and common dairy components such as saturated fat, magnesium, calcium, and vitamin D, the OR for MetS in overweight individuals decreased by 69% for those in the highest quintile for dairy intake compared to those in the lowest quintile. Among those who were not overweight, the OR for MetS decreased by 28% for those in the highest quintile compared to the lowest. Similar relationships were found for both low-fat and high-fat dairy products. A significant relationship was also found between dietary patterns with a high intake of dietary fiber and protein. Fiber intake significantly reduced the risk of MetS; for each 3 g/1000 kcal increase in fiber intake, the OR decreased by 34%. Dietary protein, however, appeared to increase the risk of MetS with a 12% increase in OR for each 1% caloric increase in protein. This relationship was only significant for protein from animal sources, no association was found for plant proteins.

The extent to which the consumption of an individual dietary component is associated with MetS is a question that still needs to be clarified. However, some studies suggest that diet quality seems to play a more important role. Baxter et al. [5] in their study concluded that no individual dietary component could be considered wholly responsible for the association of diet with MetS. Rather it is the overall quality of the diet that appears to offer protection against lifestyle disease, such as MetS [5].

5. Metabolic syndrome and hypertension: therapeutic implications

The reduction of the high cardiometabolic risk in patients with MetS is one of the main goals of interventions performed in these patients. Simple actions such as lifestyle modification measures may oppose the effect of many risk factors (lack of physical activity, overweight/obesity, and atherogenic diet). In addition, hypertensive patients usually need stricter BP control, use of antihypertensive drugs that have little impact on the metabolic profile, and quite often while taking drugs for the treatment of many other metabolic risk factors (dyslipidemia, insulin resistance, pro-thrombotic and pro-inflammatory states).

Lifestyle modifications are certainly the first measure in reaching cardiometabolic risk reduction. The main lifestyle interventions are the promotion of physical activity and weight loss with a calorie-restricted diet [63]. Calorie restriction in the range of

500–1000 kcal/day with 7–10% weight loss in 12 months and regular aerobic exercise of 30–45 minutes daily are the minimal requirements for long-term effectiveness.

Although high caloric restriction diets have not shown long-term benefits in patients with MetS, more intense regular physical activity programs have proven to offer additional cardiovascular benefits and help maintain weight loss. Lifestyle modifications have also favorable effects on BP and lipid profile and decrease the incidence of new-onset diabetes [64]. Furthermore, more recent evidence also suggests a long-term effect on reduction in both cardiovascular morbidity and mortality [65].

Additional lifestyle modifications also have been pointed out to have a positive effect on specific cardiovascular risk factors and should be encouraged in specific patients. Reduction of salt intake and alcohol consumption has a moderate effect on BP lowering, which is improved in combination with weight loss and physical activity increase [66]. Moreover, a dietary pattern rich in vegetables, fruits, and low-fat dairy products (e.g., the dietary approaches to stop hypertension [DASH] diet) substantially lowers BP in comparison with the standard American diet [67]. The MD, which is equally rich in fruits, vegetables, fish, and olive oil, also has a favorable impact on dyslipidemia in patients with MetS [68].

Maintenance of lifestyle modifications needs counseling and, for many individuals, may find it difficult in the long term. For this reason, the gradual introduction of drugs for the treatment of BP, dyslipidemia, insulin resistance, and obesity may be required to lower their cardiometabolic risk [69].

The appropriate antihypertensive treatment in MetS has not yet been established [70]. However, the choice of an antihypertensive class should be made after taking into account possible effects on glucose and lipid metabolism, as well as specific adverse events or contraindications.

No comparative studies are available on the different antihypertensive drug classes in people with HTN and MetS. Taking into account the high risk of developing new-onset diabetes in these patients as a component of cardiometabolic risk, the choice of antihypertensive treatment should not ignore this additional risk. Some international guidelines recommend diuretics as the first-choice therapy for hypertensive patients, without a compelling indication for other antihypertensive classes. However, it has been reported that diuretics increase the risk of new-onset diabetes by 23% [71]. Conversely, calcium-channel blockers (CCBs) and, especially, renin-angiotensin system blockers (ARBs and ACE inhibitors) lower this risk (33% with ACE inhibitors and 43% with ARBs). These differences are probably even more accentuated in the specific subgroup of patients with MetS. Therefore, it looks like plausible that primary antihypertensive treatment in patients with HTN, MetS, and high cardiometabolic risk should focus on inhibition of the renin-angiotensin system with either ACE inhibitors or ARBs.

More evidence comes from comparative studies of antihypertensive drugs that included an important proportion of diabetic individuals, most of them with MetS. In this regard, the Appropriate Blood pressure Control in Diabetes (ABCD) study [72] compared antihypertensive treatment based on the ACE inhibitor enalapril or CCB nisoldipine in the subgroup of hypertensive patients with diabetes. The study was prematurely stopped due to the statistical differences in the number of myocardial infarctions that favored the enalapril group in comparison with nisoldipine.

Patients with HTN and MetS, especially those with type 2 diabetes, are often less responsive to the effects of antihypertensive drugs and may require drug combinations to achieve BP control. Although some studies have demonstrated the benefits of using diuretics in combination with ACE inhibitors [73] or ARBs [74] in patients with diabetes, two comparative studies (Avoiding Cardiovascular Events through Combination Therapy in Patients Living with Systolic Hypertension [ACCOMPLISH] and Anglo Scandinavian Cardiac Outcome Trial [ASCOT]) suggest that combination of ARB with CCB could be a better option for HTN treatment in these patients.

The ASCOT study [75] compared antihypertensive treatment based on the CCB amlodipine with the addition of the ACE inhibitor perindopril in most patients against the beta-blocker atenolol with the addition of a thiazide diuretic, also in most patients. The study was prematurely stopped due to a consistent benefit of the ACE inhibitor plus CCB. More than 5,000 patients with diabetes were enrolled in ASCOT, and particular analysis of this cohort showed that the benefits of the combination of amlodipine and perindopril were also maintained in those patients with diabetes [76].

The ACCOMPLISH study [77] also compared two combinations of antihypertensive drugs in high-risk patients with HTN. Patients were treated with either the combination of the ACE inhibitor (benazepril) and CCB (amlodipine) or with benazepril plus hydrochlorothiazide. The percentage of diabetic patients in this study was around 60%. The main results showed a 20% reduction in the primary end point (composite of death from cardiovascular causes, nonfatal stroke, nonfatal myocardial infarction, resuscitation after sudden cardiac arrest, hospitalization for angina, and coronary revascularization) in the group of patients treated with benazepril plus amlodipine. The subgroup analyses did not find differences in the results in patients with or without diabetes.

Evidence to support the preference for ACE inhibitors or ARBs in the treatment of patients with MetS is lacking. The ONgoing Telmisartan alone and in combination with Ramipril Global Endpoint Trial (ONTARGET) [78] compared the ARBs (telmisartan) with ACE inhibitors (ramipril) in patients at high risk of cardiovascular events and around 30% of them were diabetic. The study found no difference in rates of cardiovascular events between the groups.

Normotensive patients with MetS often have BP levels in the prehypertension range (systolic 130–139 mm Hg and/or diastolic 85–89 mm Hg). Particular dietary interventions, such as sodium restriction or intake reduction or the adoption of the DASH diet, in addition to calorie restriction and increase in physical activity, could be useful. For diabetic patients also receiving antihypertensive treatment, ARBs are able to prevent the development of microalbuminuria in normoalbuminuric patients [79] or overt proteinuria in those with microalbuminuria [80]. For the other patients, there is no evidence for antihypertensive treatment, except that the development of HTN is prevented [81].

6. The effect of dietary patterns on blood pressure control in hypertensive patients

The benefits of different dietary patterns in reducing BP were best evaluated with the DASH diet [82] and the Nordic diet [83]. Both of these dietary patterns highlight the importance of ingestion of different combinations of healthy foods for lowering BP. Otherwise, there are little data on which types of dietary patterns are effective in lowering BP in both normotensive and hypertensive adults.

The current evidence on the beneficial effect of dietary patterns on BP in adults has been evaluated in a recent meta-analysis study that included 17 randomized controlled trials. A statistically significant reduction in BP (4.26 mm Hg in SBP and 2.38 mm Hg in DBP, respectively) was observed in this meta-analysis. For the studies that had no weight loss, sodium restrictions, or increased exercise, SBP and DBP were reduced by 4.25 and 2.27 mm Hg, respectively. A previous meta-analysis found a reduction in SBP and DBP by 6.74 and 3.59 mm Hg, respectively, from the DASH diet only [84]. The study also reported the many differences that existed between the populations that were included in the randomized controlled trials related to sex, age, intervention duration, study methodology, sample size, and difference in the combination of foods included within the different dietary patterns.

The current evidence supports that healthy dietary patterns are beneficial for BP and these include the DASH diet, MD, and Nordic diet [85]. The DASH diet mainly includes fruits, vegetables, low-fat dairy, legumes, whole grains, seeds, and low consumption of meat and saturated fat [86]. The DASH diet has been adopted in many places according to the cultural aspects such as in Australia [87], Brazil [88], and Iran [89]. Analysis of nutrient intakes and BP from the United States showed that reduced consumption of dairy products and fruit and vegetable juices was a major predictor of HTN [90]. Although the DASH diet shows positive effects from the randomized controlled trials, the studies are short-term in nature, and this may limit their generalizability as a long-term intervention.

The Nordic diet consists of foods of Nordic origin such as berries, fruits, whole grains, rapeseed oil, nuts, vegetables, fish, and low-fat dairy products. This diet when compared to a diet comprising the average nutrient intake in Nordic countries, significantly reduced 24-hour ambulatory DBP [83]. The effects of the diet, however, may not be attributed to increases in potassium or reductions in sodium because neither of these electrolytes differed between the control and intervention groups. One of the characteristics of the Nordic diet is its richness in berries.

Experimental studies models have demonstrated that the Nordic diet pattern has a beneficial effect on BP reduction [91], and in the same way, randomized controlled trials have shown that berries intake decreases BP levels [92]. Flavonoids, a type of polyphenols abundant in berries, can be the main contributing factor in the BP reduction seen with Nordic diets [93].

Further research, however, is needed on the effect of the Nordic diet on BP because studies addressing this issue are still scarce. Another dietary pattern, the MD, is usually rich in plant-based foods such as whole grains, vegetables, fruits, nuts, beans, and seeds [94]. This dietary pattern may include moderate amounts of dairy products, poultry, fish, and low amounts of red meat, although food composition may vary between different regions. In the Prevention con Dieta Mediterranean (PREDIMED) study that was carried out in Spain, the supplementation of the MD with extra virgin olive oil and with nuts lowered significantly the DBP in the MD group compared with a low-fat diet group [95]. Equally, analysis of ambulatory BP in 235 individuals of the PREDIMED study after 1 year showed significant reductions in ambulatory SBP by 4.0 and 4.3 mm Hg in the MD supplemented with extra virgin olive oil and nuts, respectively, and 1.9 mm Hg in DBP for both diets [96]. Similar effects were observed in studies of the MD carried out in Italy, where BP was also significantly lowered with this dietary pattern [97]. However, in studies from France [98] and the United States [99], no effect was found. In addition to possible differences in food and recipe composition, the study duration for these trials was less than 6 months. Because the effects of diet tend to occur over longer periods of time, a long-term follow-up may be needed to detect BP-lowering effects.

Research on the Tibetan diet that was carried out in Germany emphasized the consumption of cereals from barley, rice, corn, wheat, rye, oat, and buckwheat, and meat such as beef, mutton, chicken, roast hare, and venison [100]. Compared with the regular Western diet, there was no significant difference in BP between the Tibetan and Western diets during 12 months follow-up trial. In this regard, studies lying on the Tibetan diet are scarce and additional research is needed before conclusions on its efficacy could be done.

7. Dietary strategies for metabolic syndrome

Although the most effective dietary pattern for the management of MetS has not been established, lifestyle interventions, especially dietary habits, remain the main therapeutic strategy for its management [101]. The improvement in the quality of the foods or switching macronutrient distribution, as one of the specific dietary intervention strategies, has shown beneficial effects on MetS and individual components. Compared to the low-fat and more restricted diets, the current evidence suggests the use of the DASH diet as a strategic intervention in MetS has raised the new paradigm for MetS prevention and treatment.

An isolated nutrient dietary intervention has several limitations, and dietary counseling must be focused on the overall dietary pattern as part of MetS treatment. Recent evidence suggests the implementation of a healthy food-based dietary strategy instead of calorie or single nutrient restriction diets [102, 103]. The dietary strategies and potential health benefits for MetS and different dietary approaches are summarized in **Table 1**.

Dietary pattern	Nutritional Distribution	Improvement in MetS criteria
DASH diet	• Total fats 27% kcal/d • Saturated fats 6% kcal/d • Dietary cholesterol • CH 55% kcal/d • Proteins 18% kcal/d	• Reduction of BP (systolic and diastolic) • Reduction in BMI and waist circumference • Improvement in cardiometabolic profile • Reduction in T2DM incidence
Mediterranean diet	• 35–45% kcal/d from total fat (mainly MUFA[1], EVOO and nuts being the principal source) • 35–45% kcal/d from CH • 15–18% kcal/d from protein	• Reduction of CVD incidence and outcomes • Decreased BP (systolic and diastolic) • Inverse association with mortality • Improvements in dyslipidemia • Decreased incidence of T2DM
Nordic diet	• High content of whole-grain high-fiber products • Low in meat and processed foods	• Reduction of BP (systolic and diastolic) • Increase in HDL-c levels
Plant-based diets	• Reduction or restriction of animal-derived foods • High intake of plant-source foods • Fat profile rich in UFAs	• Reduction of BP (systolic and diastolic) • Decreased body weight and risk of obesity • Reduction of the risk of CVD • Decreased all-cause mortality • Decreased risk of T2DM

Dietary pattern	Nutritional Distribution	Improvement in MetS criteria
Low CH diets and very low CH diets (ketogenic diets)	• <50% kcal/d from carbohydrates and <10% kcal/d from CH in ketogenic diets • High protein (20–30% kcal/d) • High fat intake (30–70% kcal/d)	• Weight-loss and weight-loss maintenance • Reduction of DBP • Reduction of LDL-c and triglycerides levels • Increase in HDL-c levels • Improvements in insulin resistance • Reduction of HbA1c levels
Low-fat diet	• <30% kcal/d from total fat (<10% of saturated fat) • 15–17% kcal/d from protein • 50–60% kcal/d from CH	• Reduction of BP (systolic and diastolic) • Short-term improvement of cholesterol profile • Short-term weight loss • Reduced risk of all-cause mortality
High protein diet	• High protein (20–30% kcal/d) or 1.34–1.50 g/Kg body weight/d from protein • Low CH (40–50% kcal/d)	• Reduction of triglycerides levels
Intermittent fasting	• Fasting for a long period of time	• Weight loss • Improvements in insulin resistance • Improvements in dyslipidemia • Reduction of BP (systolic and diastolic) • Decreased risk of T2DM • Decreased risk of CVD

EVOO, extra virgin olive oil; CH, carbohydrates; CVD, cardiovascular disease; BP, blood pressure; T2DM, type 2 diabetes mellitus; DASH, Dietary Approaches to Stop Hypertension; UFAs, unsaturated fatty acids; BMI, body mass index; DBP, diastolic blood pressure; LDL-c, low-density lipoprotein cholesterol; , HDL-c, high-density lipoprotein cholesterol; HbA1c, glycated hemoglobin; MUFA, monounsaturated fatty acids.
[1]*Adapted from [101]; doi: 10.3390/nu12102983.*

Table 1.
Dietary strategies and potential health benefits for MetS[1].

8. Conclusions

The protective effects of healthy dietary patterns on MetS seem to be due to the sum of small dietary changes rather than the restriction of any single nutrient. The consumption of dietary patterns characterized by high consumption of fruit, vegetables, whole grains, legumes, seeds, nuts, fish, and dairy and low consumption of meat, sweets, and alcohol resulted in significant reductions in blood pressure.

Author details

António Gerson Bastos Francisco, Isaura da Conceição Almeida Lopes,
Amílcar Bernardo Tomé da Silva and Henrique Cotchi Simbo Muela*
Department of Physiology of Faculty of Medicine, Agostinho Neto University,
Luanda, Angola

*Address all correspondence to: henrimuela@hotmail.com

References

[1] Agodi A, Maugeri A, Kunzova S, Sochor O, Bauerova H, Kiacova N, et al. Association of dietary patterns with metabolic syndrome: results from the kardiovize brno 2030 study. Nutrients. 2018;**10**(7):898

[2] Farhangi MA, Jahangiry L, Asghari-Jafarabadi M, Najafi M. Association between dietary patterns and metabolic syndrome in a sample of Tehranian adults. Obesity Research and Clinical Practice. 2016;**10**(Suppl 1): S64-S73

[3] Aggarwal A, Aggarwal S, Sharma V. Cardiovascular risk factors in young patients of coronary artery disease: differences over a decade. Journal of Cardiovascular and Thoracic Research. 2014;**6**(3):169-173

[4] Wang J, Ruotsalainen S, Moilanen L, LepistöP,LaaksoM,KuusistoJ.Themetabolic syndrome predicts cardiovascular mortality: a 13-year follow-up study in elderly non-diabetic Finns. European Heart Journal. 2007;**28**(7):857-864

[5] Baxter AJ, Coyne T, McClintock C. Dietary patterns and metabolic syndrome - a review of epidemiologic evidence. Asia Pacific Journal of Clinical Nutrition. 2006;**15**(2):134-142

[6] Shab-Bidar S, Golzarand M, Hajimohammadi M, Mansouri S. A posteriori dietary patterns and metabolic syndrome in adults: a systematic review and meta-analysis of observational studies. Public Health Nutrition. 2018; **21**(9):1681-1692

[7] Esmaillzadeh A, Kimiagar M, Mehrabi Y, Azadbakht L, Hu FB, Willett WC. Dietary patterns, insulin resistance, and prevalence of the metabolic syndrome in women. American Journal of Clinical Nutrition. 2007;**85**(3):910-918

[8] Heidemann C, Scheidt-Nave C, Richter A, Mensink GBM. Dietary patterns are associated with cardiometabolic risk factors in a representative study population of German adults. British Journal of Nutrition. 2011;**106**(8):1253-1262

[9] Kearney PM, Whelton M, Reynolds K, Muntner P, Whelton PK, He J. Global burden of hypertension: analysis of worldwide data. Lancet. 2005;**365**(9455):217-223

[10] Mayige M, Kagaruki G, Ramaiya K, Swai A. Non communicable diseases in Tanzania: a call for urgent action. Tanzania Journal of Health Research. 2011;**13**(5 Suppl 1):378-386

[11] Naghavi M, Forouzanfar MH. Burden of non-communicable diseases in sub-Saharan Africa in 1990 and 2010: Global Burden of Diseases, Injuries, and Risk Factors Study 2010. Lancet. 2013;**381**:95

[12] Bain LKM, Myint PK, Jennings A, Lentjes MAH, Luben RN, Khaw KT, et al. The relationship between dietary magnesium intake, stroke and its major risk factors, blood pressure and cholesterol, in the EPIC-Norfolk cohort. International Journal of Cardiology. 2015;**196**:108-114

[13] Dam V, Dalmeijer GW, Vermeer C, Drummen NE, Knapen MH, van der Schouw YT, et al. Association between vitamin K and the metabolic syndrome: a 10-year follow-up study in adults. Journal of Clinical Endocrinology and Metabolism. 2015;**100**(6):2472-2479

[14] Baudrand R, Campino C, Carvajal CA, Olivieri O, Guidi G,

Faccini G, et al. High sodium intake is associated with increased glucocorticoid production, insulin resistance and metabolic syndrome. Clinical Endocrinology. 2014;**80**(5):677-684

[15] McKeown NM, Meigs JB, Liu S, Saltzman E, Wilson PWF, Jacques PF. Carbohydrate nutrition, insulin resistance, and the prevalence of the metabolic syndrome in the Framingham offspring cohort. Diabetes Care. 2004;**27**(2):538-546

[16] Hu FB. Dietary pattern analysis: a new direction in nutritional epidemiology. Current Opinion in Lipidology. 2002;**13**(1):3-9

[17] Xu H, Li X, Adams H, Kubena K, Guo S. Etiology of metabolic syndrome and dietary intervention. International Journal of Molecular Sciences. 2019;**20**(1):128

[18] Saklayen MG. The global epidemic of the metabolic syndrome. Current Hypertension Reports. 2018;**20**(2):12

[19] Grundy SM. Metabolic syndrome pandemic. Arteriosclerosis, Thrombosis, and Vascular Biology. 2008;**28**(4):629-636

[20] Ford ES, Giles WH, Mokdad AH. Increasing prevalence of the metabolic syndrome among U.S. adults. Diabetes Care. 2004;**27**(10):2444-2449

[21] Ogden CL, Carroll MD, Fryar CD, Flegal KM. Prevalence of obesity among adults and youth. United States, 2011-2014. NCHS Data Brief. 2015;**219**:1-8

[22] Mozaffarian D, Benjamin EJ, Go AS, Arnett DK, Blaha MJ, et al. Executive summary: Heart disease and stroke statistics-2016 update: A report from the American Heart Association. Circulation. 2016;**133**(4):447-454

[23] Lovre D, Mauvais-Jarvis F. Trends in prevalence of the metabolic syndrome. JAMA - Journal of the American Medical Association. 2015;**314**(9):950

[24] Akintunde AA, Ayodele OE, Akinwusi PO, Opadijo GO. Metabolic syndrome: comparison of occurrence using three definitions in hypertensive patients. Clinical Medicine and Research. 2011;**9**(1):26-31

[25] Fezeu L, Balkau B, Kengne AP, SobngwiE,MbanyaJC.Metabolicsyndrome in a sub-Saharan African setting: central obesity may be the key determinant. Atherosclerosis. 2007;**193**(1):70-76

[26] Can AS, Bersot TP. Analysis of agreement among definitions of metabolic syndrome in nondiabetic Turkish adults: a methodological study. BMC Public Health. 2007;7:353

[27] van den Hooven C, Ploemacher J, Godwin M. Metabolic syndrome in a family practice population: prevalence and clinical characteristics. Canadian Family Physician. 2006;**52**(8):982-983

[28] Clark LT, El-Atat F. Metabolic syndrome in African Americans: implications for preventing coronary heart disease. Clinical Cardiology. 2007;**30**(4):161-164

[29] Ramos RG, Olden K. The prevalence of metabolic syndrome among US women of childbearing age. American Journal of Public Health. 2008;**98**(6):1122-1127

[30] de Ferranti SD, Osganian SK. Epidemiology of paediatric metabolic syndrome and type 2 diabetes mellitus. Diabetes and Vascular Disease Research. 2007;**4**(4):285-296

[31] Chimonas T, Karagiannis A, Athyros VG, Achimastos A, Elisaf M,

Panagiotakos DB. Blood pressure levels constitute the most important determinant of the metabolic syndrome in a mediterranean population: a discrimination analysis. Metabolic Syndrome and Related Disorders. 2010;**8**(6):523-529

[32] Mancia G, Bombelli M, Corrao G, Facchetti R, Madotto F, Giannattasio C, et al. Metabolic syndrome in the Pressioni Arteriose Monitorate E Loro Associazioni (PAMELA) Study: Daily life blood pressure, cardiac damage, and prognosis. Hypertension. 2007;**49**(1):40-47

[33] Schillaci G, Pirro M, Vaudo G, Gemelli F, Marchesi S, Porcellati C, et al. Prognostic value of the metabolic syndrome in essential hypertension. Journal of the American College of Cardiology. 2004;**43**(10):1817-1822

[34] Pannier B, Thomas F, Bean K, Jégo B, Benetos A, Guize L. The metabolic syndrome: Similar deleterious impact on all-cause mortality in hypertensive and normotensive subjects. Journal of Hypertension. 2008;**26**(6):1223-1228

[35] Cuspidi C, Facchetti R, Bombelli M, Sala C, Tadic M, Grassi G, et al. Risk of new-onsetmetabolic syndrome associated with white-coat and masked hypertension: data froma general population. Journal of Hypertension. 2018;**36**(9):1833-1839

[36] Tadewos A, Egeno T, Amsalu A. Risk factors of metabolic syndrome among hypertensive patients at Hawassa University comprehensive specialized hospital, Southern Ethiopia. BMC Cardiovascular Disorders. 2017;**17**(1):218

[37] Katsiki N, Athyros V, Karagiannis A, Mikhailidis D. Metabolic syndrome and non-cardiac vascular diseases: an update from human studies. Current Pharmaceutical Design. 2014;**20**(31):4944-4952

[38] Rochlani Y, Pothineni NV, Kovelamudi S, Mehta JL. Metabolic syndrome: pathophysiology, management, and modulation by natural compounds. Therapeutic Advances in Cardiovascular Disease. 2017;**11**(8):215-225

[39] Lembo G, Napoli R, Capaldo B, Rendina V, Iaccarino G, Volpe M, et al. Abnormal sympathetic overactivity evoked by insulin in the skeletal muscle of patients with essential hypertension. Journal of Clinical Investigation. 1992;**90**(1):24-29

[40] ter Maaten JC, Voorburg A, Heine RJ, ter Wee PM, Donker AJM, Gans ROB. Renal handling of urate and sodium during acute physiological hyperinsulinaemia in healthy subjects. Clinical Science. 1997;**92**(1):51-58

[41] Vierhapper H. Effect of exogenous insulin on blood pressure regulation in healthy and diabetic subjects. Hypertension. 1985;7(6 Pt 2):II49-II53

[42] Hall JE. Mechanisms of abnormal renal sodium handling in obesity hypertension. American Journal of Hypertension. 1997;**10**(5 Pt 2):49S-55S

[43] Reaven GM. Role of insulin resistance in human disease. Diabetes. 1988;**37**(12):1595-1607

[44] Modan M, Halkin H, Almog S, Lusky A, Eshkol A, Shefi M, et al. Hyperinsulinemia. A link between hypertension obesity and glucose intolerance. Journal of Clinical Investigation. 1985;**75**(3):809-817

[45] Muscelli EO, Saad MJ, Gontijo JA. Insulin resistance in essential hypertension. Brazilian journal of medical and biological research. 1990;**23**(12):1253-1257

[46] McGill JB, Haffner S, Rees TJ, Sowers JR, Tershakovec AM, Weber M. Progress and controversies: treating obesity and insulin resistance in the context of hypertension. Journal of Clinical Hypertension. 2009;**11**(1):36-41

[47] Ogihara T, Rakugi H, Ikegami H, Mikami H, Masuo K. Enhancement of insulin sensitivity by troglitazone lowers blood pressure in diabetic hypertensives. American Journal of Hypertension. 1995;**8**(3):316-320

[48] Sanchez RA, Masnatta LD, Pesiney C, Fischer P, Ramirez AJ. Telmisartan improves insulin resistance in high renin nonmodulating salt-sensitive hypertensives. Journal of Hypertension. 2008;**26**(12):2393-2398

[49] Umeda M, Kanda T, Murakami M. Effects of angiotensin II receptor antagonists on insulin resistance syndrome and leptin in sucrose-fed spontaneously hypertensive rats. Hypertension Research. 2003;**26**(6):485-492

[50] Hall JE, Summers RL, Brands MW, Keen H, Alonso-Galicia M. Resistance to metabolic actions of insulin and its role in hypertension. American Journal of Hypertension. 1994;**7**(8):772-788

[51] Carlyle M, Jones OB, Kuo JJ, Hall JE. Chronic cardiovascular and renal actions of leptin. Hypertension. 2002;**39**(2 Pt 2):496-501

[52] Eikelis N, Schlaich M, Aggarwal A, Kaye D, Esler M. Interactions between leptin and the human sympathetic nervous system. Hypertension. 2003;**41**(5):1072-1079

[53] Marsh AJ, Fontes MAP, Killinger S, Pawlak DB, Polson JW, Dampney RAL. Cardiovascular responses evoked by leptin acting on neurons in the ventromedial and dorsomedial hypothalamus. Hypertension. 2003;**42**(4):488-493

[54] Sierra-Honigmann MR, Nath AK,Murakami C, García-Cardeña G, Papapetropoulos A, Sessa WC, et al. Biological action of leptin as an angiogenic factor. Science. 1998;**281**(5383):1683-1646

[55] Winters B, Mo Z, Brooks-Asplund E, Kim S, Shoukas A, Li D, et al. Reduction of obesity, as induced by leptin, reverses endothelial dysfunction in obese (Lep(ob)) mice. Journal of Applied Physiology. 2000;**89**(6):2382-2390

[56] Shirasaka T, Takasaki M, Kannan H. Cardiovascular effects of leptin and orexins. American Journal of Physiology - Regulatory Integrative and Comparative Physiology. 2003;**284**(3):R639-R651

[57] Considine RV, Sinha MK, Heiman ML, Kriauciunas A, Stephens TW, Nyce MR, et al. Serum immunoreactive-leptin concentrations in normal-weight and obese humans. New England Journal of Medicine. 1996;**334**(5):292-295

[58] Alvarez GE, Beske SD, Ballard TP, Davy KP. Sympathetic neural activation in visceral obesity. Circulation. 2002;**106**(20):2533-2536

[59] Khamis AG, Mwanri AW, Senkoro M, Kreppel K, Bonfoh B, Mfinanga SG, et al. Dietary patterns, nutrient intakes and metabolic conditions among agro-pastoralists in Monduli District, Tanzania. Nutrition and Dietary Supplements. 2022;**14**:11-20

[60] Williams DEM, Prevost AT, Whichelow MJ, Cox BD, Day NE, Wareham NJ. A cross-sectional study of dietary patterns with glucose intolerance and other features of the metabolic syndrome. British Journal of Nutrition. 2000;**83**(3):257-266

[61] Wirfält E, Hedblad B, Gullberg B, Mattisson I, Andrén C, Rosander U, et al. Food patterns and components of the metabolic syndrome in men and women: a cross-sectional study within the Malmö diet and cancer cohort. American Journal of Epidemiology. 2001;**154**(12):1150-1159

[62] Pereira MA, Jacobs DR, van Horn L, Slattery ML, Kartashov AI, Ludwig DS. Dairy consumption, obesity, and the insulin resistance syndrome in young adults: the CARDIA study. Journal of the American Medical Association. 2002;**287**(16):2081-2089

[63] Klein S, Burke LE, Bray GA, Blair S, Allison DB, Pi-Sunyer X, et al. Clinical implications of obesity with specific focus on cardiovascular disease: a statement for professionals from the American Heart Association Council on Nutrition, Physical Activity, and Metabolism. Circulation. 2004;**110**(18):2952-2967

[64] Knowler WC, Barrett-Connor E, Fowler SE, Hamman RF, Lachin JM, Walker EA, et al. Reduction of the incidence of type 2 diabetes with lifestyle intervention or metformin. New England Journal of Medicine. 2022;**346**(6):393-403

[65] Cook NR, Cutler JA, Obarzanek E, Buring JE, Rexrode KM, Kumanyika SK, et al. Long term effects of dietary sodium reduction on cardiovascular disease outcomes: observational follow-up of the trials of hypertension prevention (TOHP). British Medical Journal. 2007;**334**(7599):885-888

[66] Nan X, Lu H, Wu J, Xue M, Qian Y, Wang W, et al. The interactive association between sodium intake, alcohol consumption and hypertension among elderly in northern China: A cross-sectional study. BMC Geriatrics. 2021;**21**(1):135

[67] Sacks FM, Svetkey LP, Vollmer WM, Appel LJ, Bray GA, Harsha D, et al. Effects on blood pressure of reduced dietary sodium and the Dietary Approaches to Stop Hypertension (DASH) Diet. New England Journal of Medicine. 2001;**344**(1):3-10

[68] Knoops KTB, de Groot LCPGM, Kromhout D, Perrin AE, Moreiras-Varela O, Menotti A, et al. Mediterranean diet, lifestyle factors, and 10-year mortality in elderly European men and women: the HALE project. Journal of the American Medical Association. 2004;**292**(12):1433-1439

[69] de la Sierra A, Ruilope LM. Management of cardiovascular risk factors in patients with metabolic syndrome. Cardiovascular & Hematological Agents in Medicinal Chemistry. 2007;**5**(3):209-214

[70] Katsimardou A, Imprialos K, Stavropoulos K, Sachinidis A, Doumas M, Athyros V. Hypertension in metabolic syndrome: novel insights. Current Hypertension Reviews. 2019;**16**(1):12-18

[71] Elliott WJ, Meyer PM. Incident diabetes in clinical trials of antihypertensive drugs: a network meta-analysis. Lancet. 2007;**369**(9557):201-207

[72] Estacio RO, Jeffers BW, Hiatt WR, Biggerstaff SL, Gifford N, Schrier RW. The Effect of Nisoldipine as compared with Enalapril on cardiovascular outcomes in patients with non-insulin-dependent diabetes and hypertension. New England Journal of Medicine. 1998;**338**(10):645-652

[73] Patel A, ADVANCE Collaborative Group, MacMahon S, Chajmers J,

Neal B, Woodwars M, et al. Effects of a fixed combination of perindopril and indapamide on macrovascular and microvascular outcomes in patients with type 2 diabetes mellitus (the ADVANCE trial): A randomised controlled trial. Lancet. 2007;**370**(9590):829-840

[74] Lindholm LH, Ibsen H, Dahlöf B, Devereux RB, Beevers G, de Faire U, et al. Cardiovascular morbidity and mortality in patients with diabetes in the Losartan Intervention For Endpoint reduction in hypertension study (LIFE): a randomised trial against atenolol. Lancet. 2002;**359**(9311):1004-1010

[75] Dahlöf B, Sever PS, Poulter NR, Wedel H, Beevers DG, Caulfield M, et al. Prevention of cardiovascular events with an antihypertensive regimen of amlodipine adding perindopril as required versus atenolol adding bendroflumethiazide as required, in the Anglo-Scandinavian Cardiac Outcomes Trial-Blood Pressure Lowering Arm (ASCOT-BPLA): a multicentre randomised controlled trial. Lancet. 2005;**366**(9489):895-906

[76] Östergren J, Poulter NR, Sever PS, Dahlöf B, Wedel H, Beevers G, et al. The Anglo-Scandinavian Cardiac Outcomes Trial: blood pressure-lowering limb: effects in patients with type II diabetes. Journal of Hypertension. 2008;**26**(11):2103-2111

[77] Jamerson K, Weber MA, Bakris GL, Dahlöf B, Pitt B, Shi V, et al. Benazepril plus amlodipine or hydrochlorothiazide for hypertension in high-risk patients. New England Journal of Medicine. 2008;**359**(23):2417-2428

[78] Baptiste PJ, Wong AYS, Schultze A, Cunnington M, Mann JFE, Clase C, et al. Effects of ACE inhibitors and angiotensin receptor blockers: protocol for a UK cohort study using routinely collected electronic health records with validation against the ONTARGET trial. BMJ Open. 2022;**12**(3):e051907

[79] Remuzzi G, Macia M, Ruggenenti P. Prevention and treatment of diabetic renal disease in type 2 diabetes: the BENEDICT study. Journal of the American Society of Nephrology. 2006;**17**(4 Suppl 2):S90-S97

[80] Parving HH, Lehnert H, Bröchner-Mortensen J, Gomis R, Andersen S, Arner P. The effect of Irbesartan on the development of diabctic ncphropathy in patients with type 2 diabetes. New England Journal of Medicine. 2001;**345**(12):870-880

[81] Julius S, Nesbitt SD, Egan BM, Weber MA, Michelson EL, Kaciroti N, et al. Feasibility of treating prehypertension with an angiotensin-receptor blocker. New England Journal of Medicine. 2006;**354**(16):1685-1697

[82] Appel LJ, Moore TJ, Obarzanek E, Vollmer WM, Svetkey LP, Sacks FM, et al. A clinical trial of the effects of dietary patterns on blood pressure. New England Journal of Medicine. 1997;**336**(16):1117-1124

[83] Uusitupa M, Hermansen K, Savolainen MJ, Schwab U, Kolehmainen M, Brader L, et al. Effects of an isocaloric healthy Nordic diet on insulin sensitivity, lipid profile and inflammation markers in metabolic syndrome - a randomized study (SYSDIET). Journal of Internal Medicine. 2013;**274**(1):52-66

[84] Saneei P, Salehi-Abargouei A, Esmaillzadeh A, Azadbakht L. Influence of Dietary Approaches to Stop Hypertension (DASH) diet on blood pressure: a systematic review and meta-analysis on randomized controlled trials.

Nutrition, Metabolism and Cardiovascular Diseases. 2014;**24**(12):1253-1261

[85] Ndanuko RN, Tapsell LC, Charlton KE, Neale EP, Batterham MJ. Dietary patterns and blood pressure in adults: a systematic review and meta-analysis of randomized controlled trials. Advances. Nutrition. 2016;**7**(1):76-89

[86] Moore TJ, Vollmer WM, Appel LJ, Sacks FM, Svetkey LP, Vogt TM, et al. Effect of dietary patterns on ambulatory blood pressure: results from the dietary approaches to Stop Hypertension (DASH) Trial. Hypertension. 1999;**34**(3):472-477

[87] Nowson CA, Wattanapenpaiboon N, Pachett A. Low-sodium dietary approaches to stop hypertension-type diet including lean red meat lowers blood pressure in postmenopausal women. Nutrition Research. 2009;**29**(1):8-18

[88] Lima STRM, de Souza BDSN, França AKT, Salgado Filho N, Sichieri R. Dietary approach to hypertension based on low glycaemic index and principles of DASH (Dietary Approaches to Stop Hypertension): a randomised trial in a primary care service. British Journal of Nutrition. 2013;**110**(8):1472-1279

[89] Azadbakht L, Fard NRP, Karimi M, Baghaei MH, Surkan PJ, Rahimi M, et al. Effects of the Dietary Approaches to Stop Hypertension (DASH) eating plan on cardiovascular risks among type 2 diabetic patients: a randomized crossover clinical trial. Diabetes Care. 2011;**34**(1):55-57

[90] McCarron DA, Morris CD, Henry HJ, Stanton JL. Blood pressure and nutrient intake in the United States. Science. 1984;**224**(4656):1392-1398

[91] Mykkänen OT, Huotari A, Herzig KH, Dunlop TW, Mykkänen H, Kirjavainen PV. Wild blueberries (vaccinium myrtillus) alleviate inflammation and hypertension associated with developing obesity in mice fed with a high-fat diet. PLoS ONE. 2014;**9**(12):e114790

[92] Basu A, Du M, Leyva MJ, Sanchez K, Betts NM, Wu M, et al. Blueberries decrease cardiovascular risk factors in obese men and women with metabolic syndrome. Journal of Nutrition. 2010;**140**(9):1582-1587

[93] Wightman JD, Heuberger RA. Effect of grape and other berries on cardiovascular health. Journal of the Science of Food and Agriculture. 2015;**95**(8):1584-1597

[94] Serra-Majem L, Roman B, Estruch R. Scientific evidence of interventions using the Mediterranean diet: a systematic review. Nutrition Reviews. 2006;**64** (2 Pt 2):S27-S47

[95] Toledo E, Hu FB, Estruch R, Buil-Cosiales P, Corella D, Salas-Salvadó J, et al. Effect of the Mediterranean diet on blood pressure in the PREDIMED trial: results from a randomized controlled trial. BMC Medicine. 2013;**11**(1):207

[96] Doménech M, Roman P, Lapetra J, García De La Corte FJ, Sala-Vila A, de La Torre R, et al. Mediterranean diet reduces 24-hour ambulatory blood pressure, blood glucose, and lipids: one-year randomized, clinical trial. Hypertension. 2014;**64**(1):69-76

[97] Esposito K, Marfella R, Ciotola M, di Palo C, Giugliano F, Giugliano G, et al. Effect of a Mediterranean-style diet on endothelial dysfunction and markers of vascular inflammation in the metabolic syndrome: a randomized trial. Journal of the American Medical Association. 2004;**292**(12):1440-1446

[98] Vincent-Baudry S, Defoort C, Gerber M, Bernard MC, Verger P, Helal O, et al. The Medi-RIVAGE study: reduction of cardiovascular disease risk factors after a 3-mo intervention with a Mediterranean-type diet or a low-fat diet. American Journal of Clinical Nutrition. 2005;**82**(5):964-971

[99] Toobert DJ, Glasgow RE, Strycker LA, Barrera M, Radcliffe JL, Wander RC, et al. Biologic and quality-of-life outcomes from the Mediterranean Lifestyle Program: a randomized clinical trial. Diabetes Care. 2003;**26**(8):2288-2293

[100] von Haehling S, Stellos K, Qusar N, Gawaz M, Bigalke B. Weight reduction in patients with coronary artery disease: comparison of traditional Tibetan medicine and Western diet. International Journal of Cardiology. 2013;**168**(2):1509-1515

[101] Castro-Barquero S, Ruiz-León AM, Sierra-Pérez M, Estruch R, Casas R. Dietary strategies for metabolic syndrome: a comprehensive review. Nutrients. 2020;**12**(10):2983

[102] Mozaffarian D. Dietary and policy priorities for cardiovascular disease, diabetes, and obesity. Circulation. 2016;**133**(2):187-225

[103] Tresserra-Rimbau A, Castro-Barquero S, Vitelli-Storelli F, Becerra-Tomas N, Vázquez-Ruiz Z, Díaz-López A, et al. Associations between dietary polyphenols and type 2 diabetes in a cross-sectional analysis of the PREDIMED-Plus trial: role of body mass index and sex. Antioxidants (Basel). 2019;**8**(11):537

Chapter 4

Changes in Brain Metabolism Induced by Metabolic Challenges and Their Beneficial Roles for Brain Aging

Claudia Carvallo

Abstract

Life expectancy has been increasing globally along with the risk of developing Alzheimer's or other dementias. Diets high in saturated fats, refined sugars and a sedentary lifestyle are determining factors in the development of a metabolic syndrome. These factors induce energy imbalance and dysfunctional brain metabolism, hence increasing the risk of cognitive impairment and/or dementia. A cohort study with mild cognitive impairment found that it was found that the presence of three or more components of a metabolic syndrome increased the risk of Alzheimer's. On the other hand, hyperglycemia induces glutamate excitotoxicity in neurons, β-amyloid accumulation, tau phosphorylation and oxidative stress. The present chapter will cover the dysregulation of brain metabolism during physiological and pathological aging, and how metabolic challenges such fasting, caloric restriction and ketogenic diet reverts many of the deleterious effects of brain aging, favoring energy balance and cognitive function.

Keywords: brain metabolism, aging, metabolic challenges, dementia, metabolic syndrome

1. Introduction

At the brain level, physiological aging is a natural process that can be associated with the cellular and functional impairment that precedes a decline in cognitive abilities. It is widely accepted that aging is the main contributing risk factor for the onset of dementia, such as Alzheimer's disease (AD), Parkinson's disease and Huntington's disease that trigger pathological aging [1]. Studies suggest that brain aging has considerable interindividual variability [2]. Elucidating the possible genetic and/or environmental factors that can determine these differences seems to be a key point to understand why individuals may or may not trigger cognitive impairment and/or dementia. In 2015, the estimated number of people with dementia was 50 million, and the figure is projected to reach 82 million in 2030 [3]. The total cost of dementia worldwide was estimated at US$ 818 billion, which is equivalent to 1 .1% of world gross domestic product (GDP) [4], evolving into a relevant problem in global public health. A genetic analysis based on a cohort study suggested that about 75% has cognitive ability variations from childhood to old age due to environmental factors [5]. Nowadays, diets high in saturated fats, refined sugars and a sedentary lifestyle are determining factors in the development of a metabolic syndrome (MetS) such as obesity, hyperglycemia, dyslipidemia, type 2 diabetes and hypertension [6]. These factors induce an impact on various systems, including the central nervous system, thus increasing the risk of cognitive impairment and/or disorders associated with dementia [7].

Evidence shows the association between MetS and dementia, where subjects with MetS are 11.48 times more likely to develop AD compared to those without a metabolic syndrome [8]. A study carried out in China on a cohort with mild cognitive impairment found that the presence of three or more components of a metabolic syndrome increased fourfold the risk of Alzheimer's and two times only with the presence of diabetes [9]. Similarly, several studies on patient cohorts have shown that other MetS components such as abdominal obesity, hypercholesterolemia and hypertension were risk predictors of cognitive impairment and AD [10].

An explanation about the connection between a metabolic syndrome and dementias can be found in some studies. For example, type 2 diabetes can trigger Alzheimer's through hyperglycemia, which induces glutamate excitotoxicity in neurons; Furthermore, insulin resistance can contribute to β-amyloid accumulation, tau phosphorylation, oxidative stress, the formation of advanced glycation end products (AGEs) and apoptosis [11].

As life expectancy increases, the population is exposed to risk factors for longer periods of time, which may further increase the likelihood of developing dementia. In this regard, there is an increasing demand for strategies aimed at reversing the consequences of aging and its risk factors over cognitive impairment and/or dementia.

Glucose becomes the main energy demand for the brain during development. However, as time goes by, the risk of suffering from an altered energy metabolism due to the exclusive dependence on this substrate increases the pathophysiological context in the brain [12]. On the other hand, the existence of alternative energy substrates such as lactate [13] or ketone bodies [14, 15] may be beneficial for brain metabolism, thus reversing the consequences of cognitive impairment [16–18]. Lifestyles that include nutrition-based bioenergetic challenges such as caloric restriction, fasting, and ketogenic diet favor β-oxidation to produce ketone bodies that enhance synaptic plasticity, which correlates with the recovery of cognitive processes such as learning and memory [19, 20].

This chapter will study the changes in brain metabolism induced by substrates such as glucose, lactate, and ketone bodies in the context of physiological and pathological aging. Further discussion will focus on how nutritional interventions operate as metabolic modulators and neuroprotectors during physiological and pathological aging. The main interest of this section is to position the brain energy metabolism as an "energy switch" that determines the switch between physiological aging and pathological aging.

2. Brain energy metabolism: the key to the treatment of cognitive impairment and/or dementia

The human brain represents ~2% of total body mass and is the largest source of energy consumption, accounting for more than 20% of total oxygen metabolism [21], where neurons are estimated to consume between 75% and 80% of the energy produced in the brain [22]. This energy is primarily used at the synapse and a large proportion is spent on restoring neuronal membrane potentials after depolarization [23]. Therefore, normal brain function requires metabolic regulation from a single synapse level to a regional level. Neurons can use the following substrates as energy fuel: glucose, lactate, acetoacetate (AcAc) and β-hydroxybutyrate (βHB).

2.1 Cerebral glucose metabolism in physiological and pathological aging

Glucose uptake by the brain primarily starts at the blood-brain barrier (BBB). The BBB is made up of endothelial cells interconnected by tight junctions that inhibit the entry of water-soluble molecules. Passive diffusion is limited to gases and small nonpolar lipids. The rest of the nutrients need glucose transporters and monocarboxylate transporters [24, 25].

In neurons, glucose enters the cell via glucose transporter 3 (GLUT3), which is phosphorylated by hexokinase (HK) to glucose-6-phosphate (G6P) [26], which is then routed into the glycolytic pathway and the pentose phosphate pathway (PPP) [27]. The product of glycolysis is pyruvate that enters the mitochondria were metabolized through the tricarboxylic acid (TCA) cycle and oxidative phosphorylation in the electron transport chain (ETC), generating between 30 and 36 molecules of adenosine 5′-triphosphate (ATP). Pyruvate can also be generated from lactate dehydrogenase 1 (LDH1)-dependent conversion of lactate. In PPP, G6P is converted into 6-phosphogluconate (6PG) which is converted into ribulose-5-phosphate (R5P), with the production of reduced nicotinamide adenine dinucleotide phosphate (NADPH). NADPH is used to regenerate oxidized antioxidants such as glutathione (GSH) and thioredoxin. Neurons are unable to store glucose as glycogen due to constitutive degradation of glycogen synthase (GS) through glycogen synthase kinase 3 (GSK3) phosphorylation and ubiquitin-dependent proteasomal digestion mediated by the malin-laforin complex [28].

There is an astrocyte neuronal coupling where in astrocytes, glucose enters through glucose transporter 1 (GLUT1) and is preferentially stored as glycogen and metabolized through glycolysis. The generated pyruvate is converted into lactate by the expression of lactate dehydrogenase 5 (LDH5) and the inhibition of pyruvate dehydrogenase (PDH)-dependent pyruvate dehydrogenase kinase 4 (PDK4). The presence of 6-phosphofructo-2-kinase/fructose-2,6-bisphosphatase 3 (Pfkfb3) allows astrocytes to generate fructose-2,6-bisphosphate (F2, 6P) which acts as an allosteric modulator of Phosphofructokinase (PKF1) thereby enhancing glycolysis [29].

Many factors likely contribute to age-dependent brain hypometabolism. Studies, for example, show that there is higher BBB permeability in seniors, which may induce a lower intake of nutrients to the neuron and a larger accumulation of proteins such as fibrinogen, immunoglobulins, albumin, thrombin, blood hemoglobin and immune cell infiltration that may produce inflammation [30, 31]. On the other hand, studies on humans and animals show a reduced expression of glucose transporters in the brain with aging [32], as well as changes in the expression of key enzymes involved in glycolysis and oxidative phosphorylation [33].

Approximately 40% of healthy people over the age of 65 experience impairment in different cognitive domains such as working memory, spatial memory, episodic memory, and processing speed [34, 35], which is consistent with a gradual decrease in energy demand as aging progresses [36].

Functional neuroimaging studies have shown that glucose hypometabolism and mitochondrial dysfunction are early indicators of age-related functional changes during normal brain aging. Positron emission tomography (PET) analyzes with 2-[18F] fluoro-2-deoxy-D-glucose (FDG) in human subjects between the ages of 50-80 have revealed age-related decreases in glucose utilization in cortical and hippocampal regions [37]. This 14-year longitudinal study demonstrated that glucose hypometabolism can be observed decades before cognitive impairment becomes even more apparent. On the other hand, NAD levels are determinant of mitochondrial function and ATP production [38]. Studies on normal seniors show increased levels of NADH, with reduced levels of NAD and total NAD [39].

Thus, problems metabolizing glucose and impaired mitochondrial function may be a prelude to cognitive impairment and/or symptoms of dementia. Mouse model studies with reduced GLUT1 levels show an age-dependent decrease in brain capillary density, reduced cerebral blood flow and glucose uptake, and increased BBB leakage [40]. These metabolic and vascular impairments precede dendritic spine loss in hippocampal neurons and its associated behavioral alterations.

Moreover, women with AD have higher levels of amyloid plaques, neurofibrillary tangles, and higher cognitive impairment (at the same stages of the disease) than men. Recent studies show that these effects may be due to an impairment of mitochondrial complex I and an accumulation of glucose-6-phosphate (hexokinase inhibitor and rate-limiting metabolite of the PPP pathway) in AD. Furthermore, studies in mitochondria of astrocytes in the cortex and hippocampus show increased complex II-dependent respiration and increased cytochrome oxidase activity and expression of both nuclear and mitochondrial electron transport chain (ETC) subunits to compensate for metabolic disturbances in AD [41]. These data altogether show an increased female susceptibility to neuronal mitochondrial dysfunction and suggest a compensation to neuronal glucose hypometabolism through the donation of reducing equivalents via succinyl-CoA, thereby feeding succinate dehydrogenase (CII) for brain energy production inducing a neuroprotective mechanism.

Consistent with a deficit in glucose metabolism, G6P accumulation has been reported to affect the enzymatic activity of hexokinase (rate-limiting step of glucose metabolism) [42]. Furthermore, G6P is the rate-limiting substrate of the PPP which is critical for NADPH generation and subsequent detoxification of oxygen free radicals [43], thus connecting glucose hypometabolism and oxidative stress commonly observed in AD.

A recent positron emission tomography (PET) study found that the spatial distribution of aerobic glycolysis correlated with Aβ deposition in individuals with AD. This result suggests a possible link between regional aerobic glycolysis and the subsequent development of AD pathology [44, 45]. In APP/PS1 mice, glucose uptake becomes increased in the cortex and hippocampus compared to control mice. Particularly, an increase in glucose uptake is near plaques rather than in Aβ-free brain tissues, suggesting that glucose uptake may compensate for Aβ deposition [46]. Furthermore, it is presumed that weakened glucose metabolism might be a more accurate marker of neuronal atrophy than Aβ accumulation itself, since it precedes the onset of clinical symptoms in AD. In clinical studies, AD patients show early and progressive reductions in glucose metabolism in cortical and hippocampal regions. In contrast, increased glucose transport to neurons can rescue the neuronal toxicity of Aβ [47]. There actually is brain glucose deficit and hypometabolism in AD patients, which may further worsen energy insufficiency and accelerate Aβ-induced neurodegeneration.

Risk factors such as MetS in adulthood are a risk indicator for impaired brain metabolism which trigger the same metabolic effects as in pre-asymptomatic patients risking Alzheimer's. Analysis of 1H magnetic resonance spectroscopy scanning in the occipital lobe of 9 healthy participants; 10 obese nondiabetic participants; and 6 poorly controlled, insulin- and metformin-treated type 2 diabetes mellitus (T2DM) it was measured the change in intracerebral glucose levels during a 2-hour hyperglycemic clamp (glucose ~220 mg/dl). The change in intracerebral glucose was significantly different across groups. Individuals with obesity and those with T2DM had significantly reduced increments in brain glucose concentrations compared with controls (healthy 1.46 ± 0.1 mmol/l vs. obese 1.06 ± 0.06 mmol/l vs. T2DM 0.71 ± 0.1 mmol/l). Individuals with poorly controlled T2DM showed a further blunting of brain glucose levels compared with obese individuals 1.46 ± 0.1 mmol/l vs. obese 1.06 ± 0.06 mmol/l vs. T2DM 0.71 ± 0.1 mmol/l). Individuals with poorly controlled T2DM showed a further blunting of brain glucose levels compared with obese individuals [48].

2.2 Brain lactate metabolism in physiological and pathological aging

Lactate trafficking among astrocytes and neurons is mainly mediated by monocarboxylate transporter 2 (MCT2), which provides lactate uptake in neurons [49], and monocarboxylate transporter 4 (MCT4), which provides lactate release from astrocytes [49]. Both transporters serve vital functions necessary for memory formation and synaptic transmission in the hippocampus [50]. In an AD model, MCT2 and lactate levels were found to be reduced in the cerebral cortex and the hippocampus [51]. Hence, the alteration of these transporters could reduce lactate uptake into the neuron, further compromising energy metabolism and inducing cognitive impairment.

Glycogen is primarily stored in astrocytes, since its accumulation in neurons can induce apoptosis, thereby increasing the probability of suffering from dementia [52, 53]. Therefore, under physiological conditions, neurons inhibit their storage across the laforin-malin complex. Laforin is an enzyme that promotes glycogen storage but, in combination with malin, it stimulates proteasomal degradation of glycogen synthase. In the hippocampus of aged animals, Laforin becomes increased five-fold compared to adult mice and could induce increased glycogen synthesis in aged animals, which would be detrimental to neurons [54, 55].

In order to meet the energy demand of the brain, the system can generate more efficient compensatory mechanisms for quick energy production by either reducing the number of transporters in neurons or increasing the number of transporters in astrocytes.

In a study using proteomics, immunofluorescence, and qPCR in aged animals, glycogen phosphorylase (PYG), glycogen-degrading enzyme, was found to have increased its activity in hippocampal neurons, leading to a decrease in memory consolidation [56]. On the other hand, a decreased glycolytic capacity of astrocytes, along with a decrease in the number of suitable transporters for lactate secretion (MCT1) would balance the increased neuronal production of this compound, and the astrocytes would use the lactate produced by neurons to fuel. This could be a protective mechanism against neurodegeneration in the aged hippocampus.

Lactate is produced in neurons through neuronal lactate dehydrogenase (LDH) activity [57]. Native LDH consists of 4 LDHA or LDHB subunits assembled in all possible combinations, forming a variety of tetrameric LDH isoenzymes [57].

LDHA isoenzymes particularly favor anaerobic glycolysis, which may catalyze pyruvate to lactate, while LDHB isoenzymes mostly catalyze the conversion of lactate to pyruvate [58]. Studies shows that neuronal LDHA and LDHB are reduced, and that reduced levels of neuronal LDHB are more evident than neuronal LDHA in APP/PS1 mice. Meanwhile, the neuronal LDHA/LDHB ratio is increased in APP/PS1 mice compared to control mice.

On basis of these data, reduced expression of MCT2 and MCT4 is suggested to possibly prevent lactate transport from astrocytes to neurons. Consequently, neurons become lactate deficient. Also, reduced brain lactate levels further aggravate energy deficiency in neurons. Neurons can increase neuronal LDHA/LDHB ratio to favor lactate production and partially alleviate their lack of energy substrate. Nevertheless, this compensatory enzyme modification is still insufficient to compensate for energy deficiency in neurons.

Studies in human brain cortex show that lactate could replace glucose to support respiration under basal conditions and during electrical stimulation [59]. Neurons in vitro prefer lactate over glucose when both substrates are provided [60]. In vivo studies demonstrate the existence of a metabolic coupling between astrocytes and neurons where a lactate gradient from astrocytes to neurons occurs [61]. Pharmacological inhibition of MCT2 irreversibly impairs long-term memory in mice [62]. Long-term memory impairment can be reversed by intrahippocampal administration of lactate—not glucose—in MCT4-deficient mice [63]. Additionally, heterozygous MCT1 knockout mice have impaired inhibitory avoidance memory [64]. All these results strongly suggest that neuronal lactate uptake is important for the recovery of long-term memories. The overall contribution of lactate to brain metabolism differs according to its availability. Studies in conscious humans have shown that, under resting conditions, lactate uptake by the brain provides about 8% of its energy needs. This percentage increases to 20% under high plasma lactate level conditions, such as during intense exercise [65]. Furthermore, under different exercise intensities, brain lactate metabolism is higher in trained subjects compared to controls. This suggests the possibility of adaptive mechanisms that allow the brain to respond to changes in substrate availability.

In a study, plasma samples were analyzed for fasting lactate to compare lean subjects, non-diabetic subjects with severe obesity, and metabolically impaired subjects. Fasting plasma lactate was elevated in obese subjects with the metabolic syndrome compared to healthy lean individuals. These data suggest that elevated lactate may be caused by an impairment in aerobic metabolism and may offer a focus assessing the severity of the metabolic syndrome [66].

2.3 Brain metabolism of ketone bodies in physiological and pathological aging

Ketone bodies such as β-hydroxybutyrate (BHB) and acetoacetate (AcAc) are recognized as essential energy substrates for the brain during development, delivering up to 30–70% of its energy requirements [67]. In the adult brain, ketone utilization is markedly reduced when being fed, but may increase under conditions of limited glucose availability, such as during fasting, starvation, low-carbohydrate/high-fat intake, and intense or prolonged exercise sessions. Under such conditions, the liver generates ketone bodies from the oxidation of fatty acids and ketogenic amino acids. Astrocytes can metabolize and deliver ketone bodies to neurons from fatty acid β-oxidation [68], however the rates of fatty acid transport are very low compared to those in the liver. In adults, the activity of ketone- metabolizing enzymes is high enough to easily allow a complete switch from glucose to ketones to meet the energy needs of the brain [69]. Because ketones are never produced in saturated concentrations, the brain's rate of utilization is strictly regulated by their concentration in blood. In fact, brain glucose utilization during ketosis has been proven to decrease by approximately 10% per millimole of plasma ketones [70].

Whenever glucose availability declines due to fasting, starvation, exercise, caloric restriction or the ketogenic diet (KD), glycogen reserves in the liver become depleted and lipolysis of triacylglycerols or diacylglycerols in adipocytes generates free fatty acids (FFAs). The liver uses these fatty acids and ketogenic amino acids such as isoleucine, tryptophan, tyrosine, leucine, lysine, phenylalanine, and threonine. FFAs are metabolized by β-oxidation to AcetylCoA, which is used to generate ketone bodies such as AcAc, BHB and acetone (AC). AC is rapidly eliminated through urine and lungs, while BHB and AcAc cross the BBB into the neuron via monocarboxylic acid transporters (MCTs). In the anabolic pathway that takes place in the cytosol, acetoacetate is converted into acetoacetyl-CoA (AcAc-CoA) by the enzyme acetoacetyl-CoA synthase (AACS). AcAc-CoA can be synthesized into acetyl-CoA to generate sterol precursors, 3- hydroxy-3-methylglutaryl-CoA (HMG-CoA) by 3-hydroxy-3-methylglutaryl-CoA synthase 1 (HMGCS 1). Acetyl-CoA produced from AcAc-CoA by cytosolic β- ketothiolase (cBKD) or from citrate by ATP-citrate lyase (ACLY), can be converted into malonyl-CoA for fatty acid synthesis. The amino acid can be synthesized using TCA cycle intermediates. Ketone oxidation occurs in mitochondria where AcAc captured or generated directly from 3 HB by 3-β-hydroxybutyrate dehydrogenase (BDH) is converted into acetyl-CoA via succinyl-CoA-3-oxoacid CoA transferase (SCOT) and mitochondrial β-ketothiolase (mBKD). Complete oxidation of AcAc produces 23 ATP molecules, while 3 HB generates 26 ATP molecules. Additionally, astrocytes have an important local reserve of βHB for neurons [71].

Studies show that these metabolic challenges (fasting, exercise, caloric restriction, or ketogenic diet) should be intermittent as they increase insulin sensitivity and increase glucose reuptake and utilization by neurons. The incorporation of glucose stimulates the release of the hormone glucagon-like peptide 1 (GLP1), which crosses the BBB and has a direct action on neurons, hence improving cognitive function [72].

3. Metabolic challenges improve cognitive function when suffering from dementia

Whereas brain glucose metabolism declines with normal aging and more severely in AD, the ability to metabolize ketone bodies becomes another form of energy substrate for the brain and remains normal in older people and AD patients [73, 74]. Several clinical studies in aging with cognitive impairment or AD show how metabolic interventions can improve cognitive processing and possibly mitigate the effects of AD disease.

A cohort study in 70.1 (± 6.2) years patients and educational level 15.3 (± 2.8) years with cognitively impaired were given an additional 50% calories while another group consumed just 20 g of carbohydrates per day to maintain ketosis for 6 weeks. The group that held a lower caloric consumption had a higher intake of fat and protein (a typical KD). This group increased learning and memory, and their urine ketones increased by 5.4 mg/dl [75]. Researchers found that ketone concentrations had a significant correlation with memory performance.

A longitudinal study ran 2 caloric restriction diets to overweight and obese people for 1 year. A low-fat diet (46% carbohydrates and 30% total fat; <8% saturated fat) and a low-carbohydrate diet consisting of 20–40 g carbohydrates (4% energy) and a higher amount of fat (61% energy, 20% saturated). In addition to a reduction in weight, plasma glucose and serum insulin, working memory was significantly improved by KD intervention [76].

Several studies have suggested that ketogenic dietary interventions may slow functional cognitive impairment and the development of dementia; however, the benefit of KD-induced ketosis may be limited to those without the apolipoprotein E4 (ApoE4) variant [77]; a variant known to be associated with AD [78]. Nevertheless, a case study of a heterozygous ApoE4 71-year-old woman with metabolic syndrome and mild AD with progressive cognitive impairment showed significant improvement in memory measured by the Montreal Cognitive Assessment (MoCA) after 10 weeks of KD. The intervention was aimed at maintaining plasma ketones between 0.5 and 2.0 mg/dl while also doing physical and mental exercises [79]. Similarly, an obese heterozygous ApoE4 68-year-old man with mild AD and type 2 diabetes mellitus showed improvement on the MoCA scale, which represented an AD regression after 10 weeks of KD. In the latter case, a hybrid KD approach with time-restricted intermittent fasting (IF) was applied 3 days a week [80]. In both cases, improvements in various metabolic parameters such as glucose, glycosylated hemoglobin, insulin and lipid profile were documented [79, 80]. Even though multiple elements might have contributed to the cognitive improvements observed, these case studies have provided groundbreaking evidence of the potential to delay or reverse mild cognitive impairment from progressing to AD through ketogenic dietary interventions, even in ApoE4+ cases.

In view of pathological aging such as Alzheimer's, mitochondria isolated from animal models and Alzheimer's patients show reduced enzymatic activity of the cytochrome C oxidase complex (ETC IV) [81] at the cellular level, as well as decreased oxidative respiration and progressive accumulation of Aβ in the mitochondria of neurons [82]. Both metabolic dysfunction and mitochondrial Aβ accumulation appear to occur early in disease progression before the onset of amyloid plaque formation [83]. This suggests that early metabolic dysfunction is a key process in Alzheimer's progression and a potential target for therapeutic intervention.

An interesting nutritional strategy would be to improve the quality of fatty acids with medium chain fatty acids (LCFA) that are directly absorbed into the portal vein instead of the lymphatic system. Caprylic acid (C8) and capric acid (C10), medium chain fatty acids (MCFAs), are most ketogenic, which can be found in coconut oil and palm kernel oil [84]. Nevertheless, the concentration of these lipids is relatively low in coconut oil interventions, as they only raise levels of ketones slightly ~0.6 mM [84, 85].

Another alternative to the ketogenic diet is the ingestion of exogenous ketone esters and salts, which significantly increase ketone levels to >1 mM after ingestion, where ketone ester is the most potent in increasing circulating ketones even while consuming regular meals [86, 87]. Ketone salts often consist of a mixture of BHB D and L isoforms, although the metabolic contribution of L isoform is poorly understood. All three approaches (ketogenic diet, MCFA and exogenous ketone bodies) have been used in studies of neurodegenerative diseases, where MCFA becomes the most employed one. It is worth mentioning that MCFAs may have neuroprotective effects that are unrelated to ketonemia, as MCFAs can cross the blood-brain barrier (BBB) and work as substrates for energy metabolism [88]. Studies also establish that MCFA, capric acid, may have the ability to improve mitochondrial function and reduce neuronal hyperactivity, which is often observed in AD [88].

A study on 39 subjects 63-year-old with mild cognitive impairment were supplemented twice daily for 6 months with 15 g of MCFA. Participants showed an improvement in different cognitive domains, including episodic memory and executive function compared to 44 subjects with a non-ketogenic placebo. A marked increase in plasma ketones was observed only in those assigned MCFA, and this increase was directly and significantly correlated with cognitive improvements.

Another study on subjects with cognitive impairment were given 56 g of MCFA oil or a placebo (canola oil) for 6 months. Study subjects assigned to placebo reflected no changes in BHB levels or cognitive functions. Nevertheless, subjects who were administered MCFA oil as well as, one subject lacking the ApoE4 gene, showed an increase in BHB levels compared to baseline, which decreased over the following weeks. This was different from the other subject who had the ApoE gene, as he maintained this BHB increase throughout the study period. As for cognition, both subjects showed improvements in this sense, as measured by the Alzheimer's Disease Assessment Cognitive Subscale (ADAS-Cog); however, the ApoE4- negative subject showed a greater improvement.

A study on people with very mild, mild, and moderate AD showed cognitive improvement in the Mini-Mental State Examination Scale (MMSE) and ADAS-Cog after 3 months of being supplemented with an MCFA. However, this improvement in cognitive function did not persist after the dietary intervention ended. These findings suggest that efficacy depends on administration time. In another study on AD subjects, they were given 20 g of MCFA for 3 months, which led to improvements in working memory, short-term memory, and processing speed.

4. Conclusion and future directions

Brain hypometabolism of glucose and lactate to be altered long before the onset of Alzheimer's disease. Moreover, risk factors such as MetS in adulthood are a risk indicator for impaired brain metabolism which trigger the same metabolic effects as in pre-asymptomatic patients risking Alzheimer's. Therefore, providing more ketones to the aging brain can help it overcome progressive deficit in glucose absorption and metabolism, which delays brain energy depletion and decreases the risk of cognitive impairment and/or Alzheimer's disease.

Future challenges lie in elucidating the cellular and molecular mechanisms of nutritional therapies based on intermittent ketosis that account for the increase in synaptic plasticity, cognitive function, and resistance to neurodegeneration.

Understanding these mechanisms will contribute to the awareness of the pathophysiology of dementias and a more effective approach to their treatments.

Acknowledgements

This project was supported by ANID Grant Number SA77210016.

Conflict of interest

The author declares no conflicts of interest.

Author details

Claudia Carvallo
Centro de Investigación e Innovación en Gerontología Aplicada (CIGAP), Universidad Santo Tomás, Santiago, Chile

*Address all correspondence to: claudia.carvallo@usach.cl

References

[1] Hou Y, Dan X, Babbar M, et al. Ageing as a risk factor for neurodegenerative disease. Nature Reviews. Neurology. 2019;**15**:565-581

[2] Gallagher M, Colantuoni C, Eichenbaum H, et al. Individual differences in neurocognitive aging of the medial temporal lobe. Age (Dordrecht, Netherlands). 2006;**28**(3):221-233

[3] Prince M, Guerchet M, Prina M, WHO. The Epidemiology and Impact of Dementia: Current State and Future Trends. Geneva, Switzerland: WHO; 2015

[4] Wimo A, Guerchet M, Ali GC, Wu YT, Prina AM, Winblad B. The worldwide costs of dementia 2015 and comparisons with 2010. Alzheimer's & Dementia. 2017;**13**:1-7

[5] Wang X, Ji L, Tang Z, et al. The association of metabolic syndrome and cognitive impairment in Jidong of China: A cross-sectional study. BMC Endocrine Disorders. 2021;**21**:40

[6] Hasegawa Y, Chen SY, Sheng L, et al. Long-term effects of western diet consumption in male and female mice. Scientific Reports. 2020;**10**:14686

[7] Wang X, Ji L, Tang Z, et al. The association of metabolic syndrome and cognitive impairment in Jidong of China: A cross-sectional study. BMC Endocrine Disorders. 2021;**21**:40

[8] Kim YJ, Kim SM, Jeong DH, et al. Associations between metabolic syndrome and type of dementia: Analysis based on the National Health Insurance Service database of Gangwon province in South Korea. Diabetology and Metabolic Syndrome. 2021;**13**:4

[9] Ng TP, Feng L, Nyunt MS, Feng L, Gao Q, Lim ML, et al. Metabolic syndrome and the risk of mild cognitive impairment and progression to dementia: Follow-up of the Singapore Longitudinal Ageing Study Cohort. JAMA Neurology. 2016;**73**(4):456-463

[10] Mergenthaler P, Lindauer U, Dienel GA, Meisel A. Sugar for the brain: The role of glucose in physiological and pathological brain function. Trends in Neurosciences. 2013;**36**(10):587-597

[11] Tang F, Lane S, Korsak A, et al. Lactate-mediated glia-neuronal signalling in the mammalian brain. Nature Communications. 2014;**5**:3284

[12] Han YM, Ramprasath T, Zou MH. β-Hydroxybutyrate and its metabolic effects on age-associated pathology. Experimental & Molecular Medicine. 2020;**52**:548-555

[13] Takahashi S. Lactate and ketone bodies act as energy substrates as well as signal molecules in the brain. In: Takada A, editor. Psychology and Pathophysiological Outcomes of Eating. Hubertus Himmerich: IntechOpen; 2021

[14] Suzuki A et al. Astrocyte-neuron lactate transport is required for long-term memory formation. Cell. 2011;**144**:810-823

[15] Wilson KA, Bar S, Kapahi P. Ketones to the rescue of the starving fly. Nature Metabolism. 2022;**4**:159-160

[16] Newman LA, Korol DL, Gold PE. Lactate produced by glycogenolysis in astrocytes regulates memory processing. PLoS One. 2011;**6**(12):e28427

[17] Wilson KA, Bar S, Kapahi P. Ketones to the rescue of the starving fly. Nature Metabolism. 2022;**4**:159-160

[18] Silva B, Mantha OL, Schor J, et al. Glia fuel neurons with locally synthesized ketone bodies to sustain memory under starvation. Nature Metabolism. 2022;**4**:213-224

[19] Błaszczyk JW. Energy metabolism decline in the aging brain-pathogenesis of neurodegenerative disorders. Metabolites. 2020;**10**(11):450

[20] Oka M, Suzuki E, Asada A, Saito T, Iijima KM, Ando K. Increasing neuronal glucose uptake attenuates brain aging and promotes life span under dietary restriction in Drosophila. iScience. 2021;**21**(1):101979

[21] Harris JJ, Jolivet R, Attwell D. Synaptic energy use and supply. Neuron. 2012;**75**(5):762-777

[22] Pardridge WM. The isolated brain microvessel: A versatile experimental model of the blood-brain barrier. Frontiers in Physiology. 2020;**11**:398

[23] Bak LK, Schousboe A, Sonnewald U, Waagepetersen HS. Glucose is necessary tomaintain neurotransmitter homeostasis during synaptic activity in cultured glutama-tergic neurons. Journal of Cerebral Blood Flow and Metabolism. 2006;**26**:1285-1297

[24] Ckermann RF, Lear JL. Glycolysis-induced discordance between glucose metabolicrates measured with radiolabeled fluorodeoxyglucose and glucose. Journal of Cerebral Blood Flow Metabolism. 1989;**9**:774-785

[25] Baquer NZ, Hothersall JS, McLean P. Function and regulation of the pentose phosphate pathway in brain. Current Topics in Cellular Regulation. 1988;**29**:265-289

[26] Vilchez D, Ros S, Cifuentes D, Pujadas L, Vallès J, García-Fojeda B, et al. Mechanism suppressing glycogen synthesis in neurons and its demise in progressive myoclonus epilepsy. Nature Neuroscience. 2007;**10**(11):1407-1413

[27] Brown AM, Ransom BR. Astrocyte glycogen and brain energy metabolism. Glia. 2007;**55**(12):1263-1271

[28] Montagne A, Barnes SR, Sweeney MD, Halliday MR, Sagare AP, Zhao Z, et al. Blood-brain barrier breakdown in the aging human hippocampus. Neuron. 2015;**85**(2):296-302

[29] Rosenberg GA. Neurological diseases in relation to the blood–brain barrier. Journal of Cerebral Blood Flow and Metabolism. 2012;**32**(7):1139-1151

[30] Ding F, Yao J, Rettberg JR, Chen S, Brinton RD. Early decline in glucose transport and metabolism precedes shift to ketogenic system in female aging and Alzheimer's Mouse Brain: Implication for Bioenergetic Intervention. PLoS One. 2013;**8**(11):e79977

[31] Bowling AC, Schulz JB, Brown RH Jr, Beal MF. Superoxide dismutase activity, oxidative damage, and mitochondrial energy metabolism in familial and sporadic amyotrophic lateral sclerosis. Journal of Neurochemistry. 1993;**61**:2322-2325

[32] van Geldorp B, Heringa SM, van den Berg E, Marcel GM, Rikkert O, Biessels GJ, et al. Working memory binding and episodic memory formation in aging, mild cognitive impairment, and Alzheimer's dementia. Journal of Clinical and Experimental Neuropsychology. 2015;**37**(5):538-548

[33] Glisky EL. Changes in cognitive function in human aging. In: Riddle DR, editor. Brain Aging: Models, Methods, and Mechanisms. Boca Raton (FL): CRC Press/Taylor & Francis; 2007. Chapter 1

[34] Hoyer S. The young adult and normally aged brain. Its flow and oxidative metabolism. A review-part I. Archives of Gerontology and Geriatrics. 1982;**1**:101-116

[35] Mosconi L, De Santi S, Li J, Tsui WH, Li Y, Boppana M, et al. Hippocampal hypometabolism predicts cognitive decline from normal aging. Neurobiology of Aging. 2008;**29**:676-692

[36] Pittelli M, Felici R, Pitozzi V, Giovannelli L, Bigagli E, Cialdai F, et al. Pharmacological effects of exogenous NAD on mitochondrial bioenergetics, DNA repair, and apoptosis. Molecular Pharmacology. 2011;**80**(6):1136-1146

[37] Zhu XH, Lu M, Lee BY, Ugurbil K, Chen W. In vivo NAD assay reveals the intracellular NAD contents and redox state in healthy human brain and their age dependences. Proceedings of the National Academy of Sciences of the United States of America. 2015;**112**(9):2876-2881

[38] Zhao Z, Nelson AR, Betsholtz C, Zlokovic BV. Establishment and dysfunction of the blood-brain barrier. Cell. 2015;**163**(5):1064-1078. DOI: 10.1016/j.cell.2015.10.067

[39] Demarest T, Varma V, Estrada D, Babbar M, Basu S, Mahajan U, et al. Biological sex and DNA repair deficiency drive Alzheimer's disease via systemic metabolic remodeling and brain mitochondrial dysfunction. Acta Neuropathologica. 2020;**140**(1):25-47. DOI: 10.1007/s00401-020-02152-8

[40] Liu X, Kim CS, Kurbanov FT, Honzatko RB, Fromm HJ. Dual mechanisms for glucose 6-phosphate inhibition of human brain hexokinase. The Journal of Biological Chemistry. 1999;**274**:31155-31159

[41] Pandolfi PP, Sonati F, Rivi R, Mason P, Grosveld F, Luzzatto L. Targeted disruption of the housekeeping gene encoding glucose 6-phosphate dehydrogenase (G6PD): G6PD is dispensable for pentose synthesis but essential for defense against oxidative stress. The EMBO Journal. 1995;**14**:5209-5215

[42] Mosconi L, Tsui WH, De Santi S, et al. Reduced hippocampal metabolism in MCI and AD: Automated FDG-PET image analysis. Neurology. 2005;**64**:1860-1867

[43] Poisnel G, Hérard AS, El Tannir El Tayara N, et al. Increased regional cerebral glucose uptake in an APP/PS1 model of Alzheimer's disease. Neurobiology of Aging 2012;33:1995-2005.

[44] La Joie R, Perrotin A, Barré L, et al. Region specific hierarchy between atrophy, hypometabolism, and β-amyloid (Aβ) load in Alzheimer's disease dementia. The Journal of Neuroscience. 2012;**32**:16265-16273

[45] Niccoli T, Cabecinha M, Tillmann A. et al, Increased glucose transport into neurons rescues Aβ toxicity in drosophila. Current Biology. 2016;**26**:2550

[46] Hwang JJ, Jiang L, Hamza M, Sanchez RE, Dai F, Belfort-Deaguiar R, et al. Blunted rise in brain glucose levels during hyperglycemia in adults with obesity and T2DM. JCI Insight. 2017;**2**(20):e95913

[47] Newman LA, Korol DL, Gold PE. Lactate produced by glycogenolysis in astrocytes regulates memory processing. PLoS One. 2011;**6**(12):e28427

[48] Zhang M, Cheng X, Dang R, Zhang W, Zhang J, Yao Z. Lactate deficit in an- Alzheimer disease mouse model: The relationship with neuronal damage. Journal of Neuropathology and Experimental Neurology. 2018;**77**(12):1163-1176

[49] Riske L, Thomas RK, Baker GB, Dursun SM. Lactate in the brain: An update on its relevance to brain energy, neurons, glia and panic disorder. Therapeutic Advances in Psychopharmacology. 2017;7(2):85-89

[50] Hasel P, Dando O, Jiwaji Z, Baxter P, Todd AC, Heron S, et al. Neurons and neuronal activity control gene expression in astrocytes to regulate their development and metabolism. Nature Communications. 2017;**8**:15132

[51] Drulis-Fajdasz D, Gizak A, Wójtowicz T, Wiśniewski JR, Rakus D. Aging-associated changes in hippocampal glycogen metabolism in mice. Evidence for and against astrocyte-to-neuron lactate shuttle. Glia. 2018;**66**(7):1481-1495. DOI: 10.1002/glia.23319

[52] Mamczur P, Borsuk B, Paszko J, Sas Z, Mozrzymas J, Wiśniewski JR, et al. Astrocyte-neuron crosstalk regulates the expression and subcellular localization of carbohydrate metabolism enzymes. Glia. 2015;**63**(2):328-340

[53] Markert CL. Lactate dehydrogenase isozymes: Dissociation and recombination of subunits. Science. 1963;**140**:1329-1330

[54] Krieg AF, Rosenblum LJ, Henry JB. Lactate dehydrogenase isoenzymes: A comparison of pyruvate-to-lactate and lactate-to-pyruvate assays. Journal of Chromatography. B, Biomedical Sciences and Applications. 1967;**13**:196-203

[55] Markert C, Ursprung H. The ontogeny of isozyme patterns of lactate dehydrogenase in the mouse. Developmental Biology. 1962;**381**:363-381

[56] McIlwain H. Substances which support respiration and metabolic response to electrical impulses in human cerebral tissues. Journal of Neurology, Neurosurgery, and Psychiatry. 1953;**16**:257-266

[57] Bouzier-Sore A-K, Voisin P, Canioni P, Magistretti PJ, Pellerin L. Lactate is a preferential oxidative energy substrate overglucose for neurons in culture. Journal of Cerebral Blood Flow and Metabolism. 2003;**23**:1298-1306

[58] Mächler P, Wyss MT, Elsayed M, Stobart J, Gutierrez R, von Faber-Castell A, et al. In vivo evidence for a lactate gradient from astrocytes to neurons. Cell Metabolism. 2016;**23**:94-102

[59] Newman LA, Korol DL, Gold PE. Lactate produced by glycogenolysis in astrocytes regulates memory processing. PLoS One. 2011;**6**:e28427

[60] Suzuki A, Stern SA, Bozdagi O, Huntley GW, Walker RH, Magistretti PJ, et al. Astrocyte-neuron lactate transport is required for long- term memory formation. Cell. 2011;**144**:810-823

[61] Tadi M, Allaman I, Lengacher S, Grenningloh G, Magistretti PJ. Learninginduced gene expression in the hippocampus reveals a role of neuron—Astrocyte metabolic coupling in long term memory. PLoS One. 29 Oct 2015;**10**(10):e0141568

[62] van Hall G, Strømstad M, Rasmussen P, Jans O, Zaar M, Gam C, et al. Blood lactate is an important energy source for the human brain. Journal of Cerebral Blood Flow and Metabolism. 2009;**29**(6):1121-1129

[63] Kemppainen J, Aalto S, Fujimoto T, Kalliokoski KK, Långsjö J, Oikonen V, et al. High intensity exercise decreases global brain glucose uptake in humans. The Journal of Physiology. 2005;**568**:323-332

[64] Lund J, Ouwens DM, Wettergreen M, Bakke SS, Thoresen GH, Aas V. Increased glycolysis and higher lactate production in hyperglycemic myotubes. Cells;**8**:1101

[65] Edmond J. Energy metabolism in developing brain cells. Canadian Journal of Physiology and Pharmacology. 1992;**70**

[66] Garfinkel D. Simulation of the Krebs cycle and closely related metabolism in perfused rat liver. II. Properties of the model. Computers and Biomedical Research. 1971;**4**(1-2):18-42

[67] LaManna JC, Salem N, Puchowicz M, et al. Ketones suppress brain glucose consumption. Advances in Experimental Medicine and Biology. 2009;**645**:301-306

[68] Courchesne-Loyer A et al. Inverse relationship between brain glucose and ketone metabolism in adults during short-term moderate dietary ketosis: A dual tracer quantitative positron emission tomography study. Journal of Cerebral Blood Flow and Metabolism. 2017;**37**:2485-2493

[69] Mattson MP, Moehl K, Ghena N, Schmaedick M, Cheng A. Intermittent metabolic switching, neuroplasticity and brain health [published correction appears]. Nature Reviews. Neuroscience. 2018;**19**(2):63-80

[70] Han Y-M, Ramprasath T, Zou M-H. β-Hydroxybutyrate and its metabolic effects on age-associated pathology. Experimental & Molecular Medicine. 2020;**52**:548-555

[71] Vandoorne T, De Bock K, Van Den Bosch L. Energy metabolism in ALS: An underappreciated opportunity? Acta Neuropathologica. 2018;**135**:489-509

[72] Krikorian R, Shidler MD, Dangelo K, Couch SC, Benoit SC, Clegg DJ. Dietary ketosis enhances memory in mild cognitive impairment. Neurobiology of Aging. 2012;**33**:425.e19-425.e27

[73] Brinkworth GD, Buckley JD, Noakes M, Clifton PM, Wilson CJ. Long-term effects of a very low-carbohydrate diet and a low-fat diet on mood and cognitive function. Archives of Internal Medicine. 2009;**169**:1873-1880

[74] Davis JJ, Fournakis N, Ellison J. Ketogenic diet for the treatment and prevention of dementia: A review. Journal of Geriatric and Psychiatry Neurology. 2020;**34**:3-10

[75] Guerreiro R, Hardy J. Genetics of Alzheimer's disease. Neurotherapeutics. 2014;**11**:732-737

[76] Morrill SJ, Gibas KJ. Ketogenic diet rescues cognition in ApoE4+ patient with mild Alzheimer's disease: A case study. Diabetes and Metabolic Syndrome: Clinical Research & Reviews. 2019;**13**:1187-1191

[77] Stoykovich S, Gibas K. APOE ε4, the door to insulin-resistant dyslipidemia and brain fog? A case study. Alzheimer's Dementia. 2019;**11**:264-269

[78] Yao J, Irwin RW, Zhao L, Nilsen J, Hamilton RT, Brinton RD. Mitochondrial bioenergetic deficit precedes Alzheimer's pathology in female mouse model of Alzheimer's disease. Proceedings of the National Academy of Sciences of the United States of America. 2009;**106**(34):14670-14675

[79] Cheng Y, Bai F. The association of tau with mitochondrial dysfunction

in Alzheimer's disease. Frontiers in Neuroscience. 2018;**12**:163

[80] Jack CR Jr, Knopman DS, Jagust WJ, Shaw LM, Aisen PS, Weiner MW, et al. Hypothetical model of dynamic biomarkers of the Alzheimer's pathological cascade. Lancet Neurology. 2010;**9**(1):119-128

[81] Vandenberghe C, St-Pierre V, Pierotti T, Fortier M, Castellano C-A, Cunnane SC. Tricaprylin alone increases plasma ketone response more than coconut oil or other medium-chain triglycerides: An Acute crossover study in healthy adults. Current Development Nutrition. 2017;**1**:e000257

[82] Courchesne-Loyer A, Lowry C-M, St-Pierre V, Vandenberghe C, Fortier M, Castellano C-A, et al. Emulsification increases the acute ketogenic effect and bioavailability of medium-chain triglycerides in humans. Current Development Nutrition. 2017;**1**:e000851

[83] Stubbs BJ, Cox PJ, Evans RD, Santer P, Miller JJ, Faull OK, et al. On the metabolism of exogenous ketones in humans. Frontiers in Physiology. 2017;**8**

[84] Soto-Mota A, Vansant H, Evans RD, Clarke K. Safety and tolerability of sustained exogenous ketosis using ketone monoester drinks for 28 days in healthy adults. Regulatory Toxicology and Pharmacology. 2019;**109**:104506

[85] Augustin K, Khabbush A, Williams S, Eaton S, Orford M, Cross JH, et al. Mechanisms of action for the medium-chain triglyceride ketogenic diet in neurological and metabolic disorders. Lancet Neurology. 2018;**17**:84-93

[86] Koppel SJ, Swerdlow RH. Neuroketotherapeutics: A modern review of a century-old therapy. Neurochemistry International. 2018;**117**:114-125

[87] Aubert A, Costalat R, Magistretti PJ, Pellerin L. Brain lactate kinetics: Modeling evidence for neuronal lactate uptake upon activation. Proceedings of the National Academy Science USA. 2005;**102**:16448-16453

[88] Morris G, Maes M, Berk M, Carvalho AF, Puri BK. Nutritional ketosis as an intervention to relieve astrogliosis: Possible therapeutic applications in the treatment of neurodegenerative and neuroprogressive disorders. European Psychiatry. 2020;**63**:e8

Chapter 5

Effectiveness of Lifestyle Interventions for Nonalcoholic Fatty Liver Disease Treatment

Abdelilah Arredouani

Abstract

The prevalence of nonalcoholic fatty liver disease (NAFLD), which affects around 25% of the world's population, has been rapidly rising along with the rate of obesity in the world. NAFLD is now the leading indicator for liver transplantation in developed countries. NAFLD is a spectrum of diseases ranging from simple steatosis to nonalcoholic steatohepatitis (NASH), which can progress to advanced fibrosis and cirrhosis, eventually culminating in hepatocellular carcinoma. NAFLD management continues to pose challenges for patients, physicians, and healthcare systems because there is presently no approved effective pharmacotherapy. The current standard of care emphasizes intensive lifestyle interventions that include calorie restriction, increased physical activity, and weight loss. Several studies have demonstrated that weight loss of 5% or more of body weight can put NAFLD into remission. However, strict compliance and long-term effort have been an issue for many NAFLD patients precisely because of the difficulty of maintaining a sustained weight reduction. This chapter discusses the evidence supporting lifestyle intervention's effectiveness in improving NAFLD and the barriers that hinder the implementation of lifestyle adjustments and behavior changes. Finally, a few tips to help overcome these barriers are briefly discussed.

Keywords: NAFLD, steatosis, lifestyle intervention, diet, exercise

1. Introduction

Nonalcoholic fatty liver disease (NAFLD) is characterized by the buildup of lipids in the hepatocytes, as evidenced by radiologic or histologic examination. NAFLD occurs without a coexisting etiology of chronic liver diseases, such as medications, alcoholism, or viral hepatitis. The spectrum of NAFLD encompasses two subtypes: nonalcoholic fatty liver (NAFL) and nonalcoholic steatohepatitis (NASH). NAFL is marked by simple mild steatosis, described as an excessive buildup of hepatic triglycerides, typically above 5% of the liver's weight. Steatosis is generally a "benign" condition, and it does not cause liver damage but can pave the way for NASH to develop if not reversed. NASH is more aggressive and develops when steatosis combines with lobular and portal inflammation and liver cell damage in the form of hepatocyte ballooning [1]. The inflammation and liver damage of NASH can cause fibrosis, or scarring, of the liver and may lead to cirrhosis, in which the liver is scarred and permanently damaged [2]. In some cases, cirrhosis can develop into hepatocellular carcinoma [3] (**Figure 1**). Clinically, it is essential to distinguish between NAFL and NASH, as most NAFLD patients have steatosis without necroinflammation or fibrosis and do not require medical therapy.

NAFLD affects about 25% of the global population [4] and up to 30% in certain regions like the Middle East and South America [5]. NASH has emerged as the Western world's fastest-growing liver transplant indication [6]. The exact etiology of NAFLD remains elusive. However, it is accepted that obesity, type 2 diabetes (T2D), dyslipidemia, and insulin resistance (IR) are its primary causes [7]. The global prevalence of NAFLD among patients with T2D is ~55.5% [8]. Conversely, NAFLD is associated with an increased risk of developing T2D [9]. It is worth noting that NAFLD can also affect lean individuals, who account for 10–15% of all NAFLD cases [10].

The pathophysiology of NAFLD is complex and implicates increased de novo fatty acid synthesis in hepatocytes and lipid retention resulting from reduced hepatocyte apolipoprotein production and β-oxidation [11]. Epidemiological, familial, and twin studies have also provided evidence for an element of heritability of NAFLD [11–13].

An increased emphasis is being placed on discovering novel medicines to prevent, treat, or cure NAFLD due to the disease's skyrocketing incidence and the resulting medical and financial burden. Notwithstanding all efforts, no NAFLD

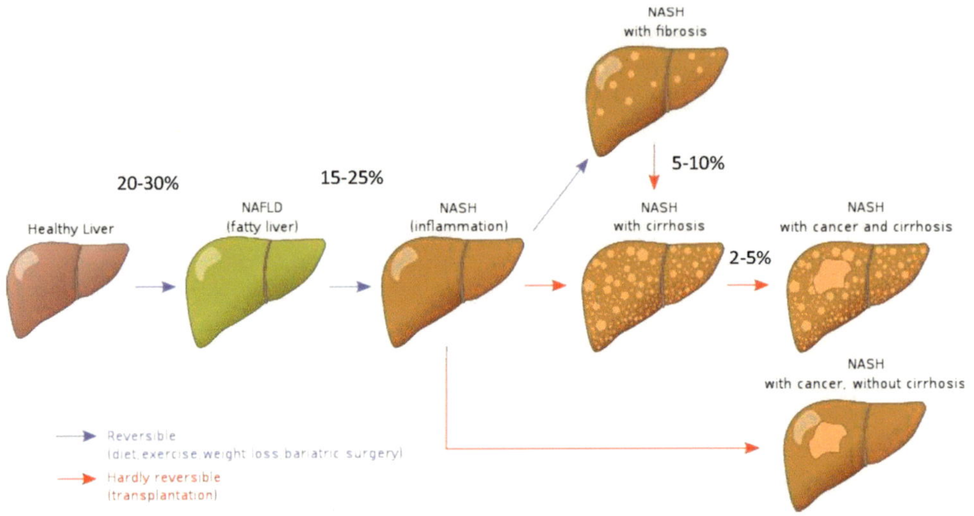

Figure 1.
The spectrum of NAFLD progression and estimated prevalence of the disease stages (adapted from https://commons.wikimedia.org/wiki/File:NAFLD_liver_progression.svg). NAFLD encompasses four stages: 1) simple steatosis (or NAFL), where fat accumulates in the hepatocytes without inflammation, ballooning, or fibrosis. Steatosis affects 20–30% of the world's population. 2) nonalcoholic steatohepatitis (NASH), where there is massive steatosis with indications of hepatocyte injury, i.e. inflammation, ballooning degeneration with or without fibrosis. Some 15–25% of steatotic patients progress to NASH. 3) within 10–20 years, some 5–10% of NASH patients may progress to liver cirrhosis, an end-stage liver disease in which most of the hepatocytes are replaced by collagen. 4) cirrhosis eventually progresses to hepatocarcinoma (HCC), where the liver is unable to regenerate and repair (liver failure), and transplantation is required. HCC affects 2–5% of cirrhotic patients. Factors that cause simple steatosis include calorie-dense Western diets, obesity, T2D, and insulin resistance. Inflammation and hepatocyte apoptosis are factors that contribute to the development of NASH. Liver fibrosis is a transitional phase of NASH that results in the development of liver cirrhosis. Steatosis and NASH/fibrosis could be reversed with lifestyle adjustments, while cirrhosis and HCC are hardly reversible.

pharmacotherapy has yet been approved [5]. At best, physicians can prescribe various medicines to manage the disorders associated with the condition, including hypertension, hypercholesterolemia, T2D, and obesity. Nowadays, weight loss remains the cornerstone treatment for NAFLD. Several randomized controlled trials (RCTs) have shown that ≥5% weight loss improved steatosis, while ≥7% weight loss improved the NAFLD activity score (NAS) [14]. Dietary interventions showed that energy restriction was crucial to improvement in liver fat and transaminase levels. Intensive lifestyle interventions (ILIs) have shown significant success in NAFLD [15]. In the sections below, the limitations of the current NAFLD treatments and the results obtained with ILI-based clinical trials will be discussed.

2. Limitations of current NAFLD treatments

NAFLD is one of the medical requirements with the greatest unmet potential for pharmacotherapeutic treatments, despite being the most common cause of chronic liver disease globally. NAFLD patients frequently have metabolic comorbidities such as obesity, hyperlipidemia, IR, and T2D [16]. Therefore, the management of NAFLD should consist of treating liver disease as well as these comorbidities. Some of the treatments that have been tried so far include dietary supplements, including polyunsaturated fatty acids (PUFAs), vitamins, and resveratrol, and drugs, including metformin, thiazolidinedione, incretin analogs, glifozines, statins, ACC, FAS, and DGAT1/2 inhibitors, obeticholic acid, SARTANS (telmisartan, valsartan, and losartan), and finally the more invasive bariatric surgery.

Supplementation with polyunsaturated fatty acids (PUFAs) was examined in the management of NAFLD, considering the promising outcomes gained by using a Mediterranean diet (MD) high in PUFAs. A meta-analysis of nine studies involving 355 participants looked at the effect of omega-3 or fish oil supplementation on NAFLD and found that, despite being extremely heterogeneous, some results showed that supplemented patients had significantly lower fatty liver [17]. n-3 PUFA supplementation dramatically reduced liver fat compared to placebo, and it also improved levels of triglycerides, total cholesterol, high-density lipoprotein, and BMI, according to a new meta-analysis comprising up to 22 RCTs and 1366 participants [18]. However, alanine transaminase (ALT), aspartate aminotransferase (AST), and γ-glutamyl transferase (GTT) levels were not significantly improved [18]. Higher blood levels of total n-6 PUFA and linoleic acid were linked to lower probabilities of developing NAFLD in middle-aged and older Finnish people, according to a recent study [19]. The exact mechanism of ω-3 PUFAs' beneficial effect on NAFLD is not fully understood. However, it might result from the combination of their transcriptional repression activity on acetyl-CoA carboxylase (ACC), fatty acid synthase (FASN), and L-pyruvate kinase, critical hepatic glycolysis, and de novo lipogenesis enzymes [20], as well as their prominent antioxidant, regenerative, and antitumor properties [21]. Despite these promising results, there is a need for well-designed RCTs which quantify the magnitude of the effect of PUFAs supplementation on liver fat as well as the quantities required to achieve a significant effect on liver fat content and improve liver enzyme levels.

Diet and exercise-related lifestyle decisions made by an individual have a major impact on NAFLD. Accordingly, research has highlighted the significance of calorie restriction and macronutrient composition in influencing illness outcomes. However, the liver is also crucial in micronutrient metabolism, and dysregulation of this metabolism may contribute to NAFLD development. Recent studies have highlighted the relation between dietary vitamins and fat accumulation in the liver [22]. A growing number of studies have linked vitamins, notably vitamin E, to NAFLD, and vitamin supplementation has been suggested as a possible therapeutic strategy in treating NAFLD [23]. Changes in the serum levels of vitamin D, vitamin B_{12}, and folate have demonstrated a high link with the severity of NAFLD, and the antioxidant activities of vitamins C and E have been credited with reducing hepatocyte injury. Several biochemical alterations in NAFLD, including the lipotoxic hepatic environment, the altered immune system, the unwarranted inflammation, the oxidative stress, the epigenetic modifications, and the gut dysbiosis, correlate to derangement in vitamins [24]. More carefully planned studies on the human population are still required to establish vitamins' effectiveness and safety as therapeutic agents, despite the attractive prospective choices to improve NAFLD management with vitamins. In fact, high doses of vitamin E were shown to be toxic and could increase the risk of cardiovascular mortality [25].

Resveratrol is a polyphenol in berries, including grapes, blueberries, and blackberries [26], and was suggested as a potential treatment option for managing NAFLD given its anti-inflammatory and antioxidant properties, as well as calorie restriction-like effects [27]. By reducing lipogenesis and inflammation, resveratrol reduces hepatic steatosis in high-fat-fed mice [28]. For treating NAFLD in humans, a 12-week supplementation of 500 mg of resveratrol and lifestyle modification was superior to lifestyle modification alone [29]. This effect was attributed partially to the attenuation of inflammatory markers and hepatocellular apoptosis. However, the number of participants was small ($n = 50$ for both arms), and studies with larger cohorts are warranted for validation.

Presently, neither the FDA nor the EMA (European Medicines Agency) has approved a medication for the treatment of NAFLD. Consequently, the agencies concur that any drug provided for therapeutic purposes for NAFLD is regarded as an off-label treatment, and that this therapeutic strategy is addressed with the patient while considering the risk/benefit ratio [30]. Some of the drugs considered relevant for NAFLD treatment are presented in **Table 1**. It is beyond this chapter's scope to discuss each drug's mechanisms of action, but the reader can find ample information in the literature, such as in [101–103].

3. Lifestyle modification in NAFLD treatment

It is commonly accepted that lifestyle variables, such as an excessive intake of calorie-dense foods and a sedentary lifestyle, are directly related to the pathophysiology of NAFLD, even though the involvement of genetic predisposition in the development of the disease cannot be eliminated. This link is demonstrated by the parallelism between the occurrence of NAFLD and obesity worldwide. Intensive lifestyle interventions, such as dietary changes and regular physical activity that led to significant weight loss, have been the mainstays of NAFLD management and treatment thus far. When successful, lifestyle modifications are far more effective at lowering fibrosis and necroinflammatory alterations in NASH than medications currently being trialed. Therefore, lifestyle modification is considered the main clinical recommendation and the initial step in managing NAFLD. The research supporting the use of lifestyle modification to treat NAFLD/NASH patients' hepatic steatosis and liver histology is examined in this section. Since long-lasting lifestyle changes and

DOI: http://dx.doi.org/10.5772/intechopen.106445

Drug action	Medication	Action on NAFLD/NASH	Limitations	References
Anti-diabetic drugs	Metformin	• Decrease in hepatic and peripheral insulin resistance • ↓Hepatic neoglucogenesis • ↓De novo lipogenesis • ↑FA oxidation	Gastrointestinal side effects including acidosis lactic acid and hepatotoxicity	[31–42]
	Thiazolidinedione	• PPAR-γ agonists • ↑ Adiponectin • ↑ β-Oxidation • ↓ Lipogenesis • ↑ Adipogenesis	Myocardial infarction + bladder cancer: drugs withdrawn from sale in France	[43–52]
	Incretin analog	• GLP-1 (liraglutide) analogs • Resolution of steatosis without the aggravation of fibrosis in NASH patients. • Improved insulin sensitivity, weight loss, and decreased DNL • OPP-IV inhibitors (sitagliptin) • Correlation between DPP-IV level and NAFLD'NASH stage • Improvement of liver function	• Lack of data and need for further studies • Little effect on =NAFLD and NASH despite improvement in liver function	[32, 33, 53–63]
SGLT2 Inhibitors	Glifozines	• Urinary glucose excretion: • Weight loss • Improvement of liver function • Improvement of liver fibrosis	• Urinary side effects include urosepsis, urogenital infections, and pyelonephritis	[49, 64–67]
Hyperlipidemia drugs	Statines	• Hepatic cholesterol synthesis via inhibition of HMGCoA reductase: improvement of hepatic fibrosis and steatosis	• Mixed results hepatotoxic potential	[68–71]
	Ezetimibe	• ↑Insulin sensitivity, • ↓Steatosis, cholesterol levels, and ALT levels	• No effects on fibrosis and hepatic inflammation	[72–74]

Drug action	Medication	Action on NAFLD/NASH	Limitations	References
Regulators of hepatic lipid metabolism	ACC inhibitors	• ↓DNL and hepatic steatosis • ↑β-Oxidation of FAs	• First-generation inhibitors associated with hypertriglyceridemia • Second-generation inhibitors: partial 5 days of DNL without reactive hypertriglyceridemia (study in progress)	[75–82]
Regulators of hepatic lipid metabolism FXR agonists	FAS inhibitors	• DNL inhibition. Effective in NAFLD and NASH	PHASE I	[48, 83–85]
	DGAT1/2 Inhibitors	• ↓DNL and hepatic steatosis • ↑β-Oxidation of FAs	• Efficacy controversial-on fibrosis DGAT1:gastrointestinal toxicity	[76, 86–88]
	OBETICHOLIC ACID	• Anti-inflammatory • Anti-fibrotic	• Atherogenic potential and pruritus	[89–97]
Antihypertensive drugs	SARTANS (telmisartan, valsartan, losartan)	• Losartan: 5 days hepatic fibrosis + necroinflammation • Valsartan: IR improvement + fibrosis • Telmisartan: IR improvement + fibrosis +↓ circulating FAs levels + steatosis	• Further studies are needed	[52, 98–100]

Table 1.
A non-exhaustive table of studies that tried different potential pharmaceuticals for the treatment of NAFLD/NASH.

weight loss are challenging to achieve [104] and unfortunately, altering one's lifestyle alone does not always succeed, the different hurdles to adopting these changes are highlighted, along with strategies to overcome them.

A number of RCTs have demonstrated that altering one's lifestyle aids individuals with NAFLD in shedding pounds, lowering liver fat content, and raising their NAFLD activity score, which is a combination of steatosis, inflammation, and hepatic ballooning and is determined by liver biopsy. In a very recent meta-analysis of 30 RTCs involving 3280 participants with proven NAFLD, Fernandez et al., [104] found that combined exercise and diet intervention leads to significant reductions in ALT, AST, and HOMA-IR (Homeostatic Model Assessment for Insulin Resistance) than diet or exercise alone. Also, Peterson and coworkers [105] reported a reversal of intrahepatic lipid in eight obese subjects following a 12-week moderately hypocaloric, very-low-fat (3%) diet (~1200 kcal/day) that led to a weight loss of only ~8 kg. Furthermore, in an RCT examining the effects of weight loss on clinical parameters of NASH, Promrat et al., [106] employed a 48-week ILI that combined diet, exercise, and behavior change, and targeting 7 to 10% weight loss, on 31 overweight/obese adults with biopsy-proven NASH. The patients were randomized in a 2:1 ratio to receive ILI or structured education (control). The change in NASH histological activity score (NAS) was the primary outcome (NAS ranges between 0 and 8) and is used to grade NAFLD: NAS $\geq$ 5 indicates NASH, and NAS $\leq$ 3 indicates no NASH [106]. In contrast to the control group, which lost 0.2% of weight after 48 weeks, patients allocated to ILI lost an average of 9.3% of their body weight. A significant correlation was observed between percent weight reduction and improvement in NAS ($r = 0.497$, $P = 0.007$). When compared to the control group (4.9 to 3.9), NAS dramatically improved in the ILI (from 4.4 to 2.0;$P = 0.05$). Compared to those who lost less than 7%, the patients who achieved the study weight loss goal significantly improved steatosis, lobular inflammation, ballooning injury, and NAS.

In an RCT undertaken by Katsagoni and coworkers in Greece [107], 63 ultrasonography-proven obese NAFLD patients with high ALT and/or GGT levels received 6 months of Mediterranean lifestyle intervention consisting of a Mediterranean diet (MD) along with guidance to increase physical activity and improve sleep habits. Compared to control patients, who received only written information for a healthy lifestyle, the Mediterranean lifestyle intervention patients showed a significant 50% reduction of ALT levels and liver stiffness after adjusting for % weight loss and baseline values. An RCT has looked at the impact of the green Mediterranean diet (GMD), which further restricts red and processed meat while enhancing green vegetables and polyphenols, on NAFLD as measured by intrahepatic fat (IHF) reduction [108]. In this 18-month study, 294 participants with abdominal obesity/dyslipidemia were divided into three weight-loss groups: healthy dietary guidelines (HDGs), MD, and green-MD, all of which included physical activity. NAFLD prevalence declined significantly to 54.8%, 47.9%, and 31.5% in HDG, MD, and GMD groups, respectively ($p = 0.012$ between groups). Even while the two MD groups experienced similar modest weight reduction, it is interesting to note that the GMD group experienced over twice as much intrahepatic fat (IHF) % loss (−38.9% proportionately) as compared to the MD and HDG groups.

In a very recent parallel, multicenter RCT, George and coworkers [109] looked at the impact of a Mediterranean diet (MD) on hepatic and metabolic outcomes in NAFLD. The 42 participants were randomized (1:1 ratio) to MD or low-fat diet (LFD) for 12 weeks. The results revealed that intrahepatic lipids and insulin resistance (measured by HOMA-IR) improved significantly within the LFD group but not within the MD group. The visceral fat was reduced significantly in both groups. It is worth noting that this RCT did not involve any physical activity, which could have improved the results. Results from a recent [110] 52-week phase IV double-blind parallel RCT comparing the effects of lifestyle and dietary intervention plus Ezetimibe to lifestyle versus dietary intervention alone (placebo) on the progression and complications of NASH revealed that Ezetimibe administered in addition to lifestyle and dietary modification failed to significantly improve the histology of NASH beyond what is achieved with lifestyle and dietary modification alone.

In a 2-year RCT, Marin-Alejandro and colleagues examined the results of two customized dietary approaches in NAFLD patients [111]. The 98 participants were divided into two groups at random: the test group received the Fatty Liver in Obesity (FLiO) diet and the control group received the American Heart Association (AHA) diet. The AHA diet is based on AHA recommendations for eating habits and lifestyle changes, and it aims to reduce body weight by at least 3–5% and as much as 10% to reduce liver disease-related necrotizing inflammation. The FLiO diet is a Mediterranean diet that has the same targets as the AHA diet and is based on a quantitively and qualitatively good distribution of macronutrients, meal frequency, dietary behavior, antioxidant capacity, and lifestyle advice. The FLiO group outperformed the AHA group at the end of the study in terms of ALT, liver stiffness, and Fatty Liver Index, among other outcomes. However, weight loss percentage attenuates these differences when the analyses were adjusted. These results demonstrate that both approaches are viable substitutes for managing NAFLD. The FLiO method, however, might offer more long-lasting advantages in terms of metabolic and hepatic characteristics. Because of the limited space, only a few RTCs that reported the positive effect of lifestyle adjustments on NAFLD are reported above. **Table 2** shows some more similar RTCs conducted in the last 2 years.

4. Barriers and facilitators to implementing a lifestyle change for NAFLD

According to the evidence outlined in the previous section, NAFLD therapy based on intensive lifestyle intervention that combines diet and exercise can be successful. However, there are numerous obstacles to the clinical implementation of lifestyle intervention. For instance, the majority, if not all, intensive lifestyle therapies designed to improve NAFLD/NASH necessitate a weight loss of at least 5% of body weight. However, weight loss is notoriously difficult to achieve and even more challenging to maintain [119]. Without weight loss maintenance, the effect of ILI will, at best, be temporary. In a prospective observational cohort study, Jimenez and coworkers [110] evaluated the influence of weight regain on the NAFLD, assessed utilizing a fibrosis score 3 years post Roux-en-Y-gastric bypass surgery. They observed that of the 90 patients examined, 35.6% had obesity recurrence and that the fibrosis score in this group was significantly higher than in the group that had no weight regain. Similar to this, Nakanishi et al., [120] recently showed that among male participants who had been diagnosed with NAFLD and had entered remission, weight gain of 1.5 kg or more and a lack of exercise were related with NAFLD recurrence. The findings of these two studies strongly indicate that maintaining a weight loss is necessary to maintain NAFLD remission.

Additionally, the success of implementing ILI for NAFLD management requires the care to be best provided by multidisciplinary teams incorporating physicians who are experts in the management of NAFLD and its comorbidities, nutritionists,

Study	Design	Number of patients	Objective	Outcome
George ES et al., [112]	Parallel multicenter RTC	42 NAFLD patients	Assess the effect of MD or LFD for 12 weeks on IHL	LFD improved IHL and insulin resistance. Significant improvements in visceral fat were seen within both groups
Montemayor S et al., [113]	Cross-sectional study	155 Ow/Ob NAFLD patients with MetS	To evaluate the impact of a tailored hypocaloric diet and increased physical exercise on IHL and NAFLD progression	Subjects with NAFLD and MetS had reduced intrahepatic fat content and liver stiffness in response to diet and exercise
Noto D et al., [114]	Double-blind RCT	40 patients with ascertained NASH	Compare Lifestyle adjustment versus ezetimibe + lifestyle	Ezetimibe + lifestyle modification is not superior in improving NAHS than lifestyle modification alone
Mascaro CM et al., [115]	Prospective cohort analysis of data obtained between baseline and 6-year parallel-group randomized trial	155 NAFLD patients with MetS	Compare the effect of 6-month CD versus MD-high meal frequency or MD + physical activity on fitness status	Lifestyle 6-month intervention with diet and regular PA improved functional fitness in patients with NAFLD and MetS
Meir AY et al., [108]	Eighteen-month randomized clinical trial	294 participants with abdominal obesity/dyslipidemia	Analyze the impact of a green-MD diet, which is low in red and processed meat and high in green vegetables and polyphenols, on NAFLD as shown by loss of IHL.	Green-MD can double IHL loss and reduce NAFLD in half compared to healthy dietary guidelines or regular MD
Jovanovic GK et al., [116]	RCT	81 obese participants	After a 6-month follow-up, assess the impact of an anti-inflammatory diet with lower energy intake on the liver health in younger persons with obesity.	The anti-inflammatory diet induced a significant improvement of liver parameters in younger adults with obesity
Marin-Alejandre BA et al., [111]	RCT	98 NAFLD patients	Evaluate the long-term effects AHA and FLiO diets on weight loss, and metabolic and hepatic outcomes in overweight/obese subjects with NAFLD	The AHA and FLiO diets were able to improve body weight and body composition, as well as the metabolic and hepatic status of participants with overweight/obesity and NAFLD within a 2-year follow-up

Study	Design	Number of patients	Objective	Outcome
Franco I et al., [117]	RCT	144 patients with moderate or severe NAFLD	Estimate the effect of two different PA programs, a low (LGIMD), and their combined effect on the NAFLD score	LGIMD + aerobic activity program was the most efficient in reducing NAFLD score when compared to CD, LGIMD, aerobic activity, aerobic activity + resistance training, and LGIMD+ aerobic activity + resistance training
Ristic-Medic D et al., [118]	RCT	24 NAFLD patients	Analyze the impact of MD and LFD on patients with NAFLD's fatty acid profiles, cardiometabolic indicators, and liver condition.	Given that it improves fatty liver and decreases saturated and increases monounsaturated and n-3 polyunsaturated fatty acid status in NAFLD patients, the MD may contribute to disease treatment even more than the LFD.

Table 2.
Some of the RTCs undertaken between 2020 and the present to assess the lifestyle modifications on NAFLD. LFD: Low-fat diet; MD: Mediterranean diet; IHL: Intrahepatic lipids; ow/Ob: Overweight/obese; CD: Conventional diet; AHA: American Heart Association; FLiO: Fatty liver in obesity; PA: Physical activity; LGIMD: Glycemic index Mediterranean diet.

educators, physical exercise coaches, as well as the patients' families. It also requires discipline, monitoring for complications, and regular laboratory assessments. The goal should be to foster an environment that promotes maintaining healthy body weight and body composition as a way of life. Another barrier to implementing ILI for NAFLD management is the lack of training necessary to deliver it among the health providers. In fact, a study by Avery et al., [121] has found a significant gap between recommendations and how clinical treatment is provided in reality. Healthcare professionals acknowledged a lack of knowledge and tools on how to successfully target lifestyle behavior change to control NAFLD over the long term and the necessity for a collaborative approach across disciplines to avoid miscommunicating with patients. Patients also supported this conclusion by reporting a severe shortage of information and support at the time of diagnosis and moving forward.

Patients must comprehend their disease to be convinced to adopt successful, long-lasting lifestyle adjustments. Impactful changes in their lifestyle habits will be hindered by their lack of knowledge of their condition and their failure to recognize the relationship between their current lifestyle choices and their disease, NAFLD, in this case. Patients must comprehend that if they make and sustain effective lifestyle adjustment, NAFLD/NASH may be curable [121].

Finally, it is important to remember that a variety of factors, including gender and reproductive status, genetics, the richness of the gut microbiota, endocrine and metabolic condition, and physical activity, may contribute to the variability of

NAFLD. Therefore, the individual patient should consider all these factors to implement an individualized lifestyle adjustment. A one-size-fits-all lifestyle adjustments plan may not be adequate for all NAFLD patients. The impact of considering NAFLD heterogeneity on the development of targeted therapies for NAFLD is crucial for the success of the intervention [120].

A variety of lifestyle adjustment strategies and behavior change counseling techniques are available for usage, some with a more robust evidence base than others for addressing each stage in the process. These methods are intended to aid healthcare professionals and doctors in guiding patients toward making informed decisions about their actions and inspiring them to take ownership of their health. For instance, using motivational interviewing techniques during consultations can help patients feel more empowered to make their own health-related decisions. Some of the practical tips to support patients to make lifestyle changes include but not limited to 1) dispelling any myths, such as the idea that alcohol is the cause of NAFLD, by describing what NAFLD is and how it may be reversed with lifestyle changes; 2) explain the link between the body weight changes and the energy balance concept; 3) set a weight loss target that is realistic, personalized, quantifiable, attainable, and relevant; 4) encourage the use of self-monitoring tools, such as routine weighing, tracking calorie consumption by keeping a daily log, wearing activity trackers, understanding nutritional labels and choosing healthier options, acquiring knowledge of how to buy for, prepare, and serve meals; 5) utilize the proper interventions, such as regular meal patterns, fewer snacking, and portion control; 6) motivate patients to join local gyms, weight management programs, and walking groups; there is evidence that diet and physical activity interventions delivered in groups are effective in promoting clinically meaningful weight loss [122].

5. Conclusion

In the absence of an approved pharmacotherapy for NAFLD, ILIs remain the cornerstone for treating the condition. Strong evidence indicates that a sustained weight loss of 5% or more of the body weight can lead to NAFLD remission in a sizable proportion of patients. From the several RTCs listed in this study, lifestyle changes based on Mediterranean diets and exercise appear to be the most successful for improving NAFLD in a significant number of patients. Additionally, considering patient heterogeneity with regard to their reaction to ILIs, i.e. creating individualized ILI, may enhance the success of the intervention in NAFLD patient subgroups. In certain resistive patients, subtle changes in the composition of the meals or in exercise intensity may be more beneficial. As the number of NAFLD patients keeps increasing, health providers must have the ability and capacity within healthcare settings to motivate and support patients to make long-lasting lifestyle behavior adjustments. More emphasis should be placed on engaging patients in a discussion about their choices concerning their care. To better tackle NAFLD, healthcare providers should set up multidisciplinary teams with different expertise, i.e. hepatology, diabetology, cardiology, obesity, nutrition, and physical education.

Implementing effective lifestyle interventions for NAFLD patients is crucial not only because of the significant disease prevalence worldwide but also because excess liver fat is a separate risk factor for the onset of cardiovascular disease and T2D [123].

Acknowledgements

The author is grateful to the Qatar Biomedical Research Institute for the continuing support.

Conflict of interest

The author declares no conflict of interest.

Author details

Abdelilah Arredouani[1,2]

1 Diabetes Research Center, Qatar Biomedical Research Institute, Hamad Bin Khalifa University, Qatar Foundation, Doha, Qatar

2 College of Health and Life Sciences, Qatar Foundation, Hamad Bin Khalifa University, Doha, Qatar

*Address all correspondence to: aarredouani@hbku.edu.qa

References

[1] Kleiner DE, Makhlouf HR. Histology of nonalcoholic fatty liver disease and nonalcoholic steatohepatitis in adults and children. Clinics in Liver Disease. 2016;**20**(2):293-312

[2] Li B, Zhang C, Zhan YT. Nonalcoholic fatty liver disease cirrhosis: A review of its epidemiology, risk factors, clinical presentation, diagnosis, management, and prognosis. Canadian Journal of Gastroenterology & Hepatology. 2018;**2018**:2784537

[3] Pinyopornpanish K et al. Hepatocellular carcinoma in nonalcoholic fatty liver disease with or without cirrhosis: A population-based study. BMC Gastroenterology. 2021;**21**(1):394

[4] Younossi ZM. Non-alcoholic fatty liver disease–a global public health perspective. Journal of Hepatology. 2019;**70**(3):531-544

[5] Younossi ZM et al. The economic and clinical burden of nonalcoholic fatty liver disease in the United States and Europe. Hepatology. 2016;**64**(5):1577-1586

[6] Burra P, Becchetti C, Germani G. NAFLD and liver transplantation: Disease burden, current management and future challenges. JHEP Reports. 2020;**2**(6):100192

[7] Ota T. Molecular mechanisms of nonalcoholic fatty liver disease (NAFLD)/nonalcoholic steatohepatitis (NASH). Advances in Experimental Medicine and Biology. 2021;**1261**:223-229

[8] Younossi ZM et al. The global epidemiology of NAFLD and NASH in patients with type 2 diabetes: A systematic review and meta-analysis. Journal of Hepatology. 2019;**71**(4):793-801

[9] Sung KC et al. Combined influence of insulin resistance, overweight/obesity, and fatty liver as risk factors for type 2 diabetes. Diabetes Care. 2012;**35**(4):717-722

[10] DiStefano JK, Gerhard GS. NAFLD in normal weight individuals. Diabetology and Metabolic Syndrome. 2022;**14**(1):45

[11] Pafili K, Roden M. Nonalcoholic fatty liver disease (NAFLD) from pathogenesis to treatment concepts in humans. Molecular Metabolism. 2021;**50**:101122

[12] Dongiovanni P, Valenti L. Genetics of nonalcoholic fatty liver disease. Metabolism. 2016;**65**(8):1026-1037

[13] Carlsson B et al. Review article: The emerging role of genetics in precision medicine for patients with non-alcoholic steatohepatitis. Alimentary Pharmacology & Therapeutics. 2020;**51**(12):1305-1320

[14] Peng L, Wang J, Li F. Weight reduction for non-alcoholic fatty liver disease. Cochrane Database of Systematic Reviews. 2011;**6**:Cd003619

[15] Dudekula A et al. Weight loss in nonalcoholic fatty liver disease patients in an ambulatory care setting is largely unsuccessful but correlates with frequency of clinic visits. PLoS One. 2014;**9**(11):e111808

[16] Chalasani N et al. The diagnosis and management of nonalcoholic fatty liver disease: Practice guidance from the American Association for the Study of Liver Diseases. Hepatology. 2018;**67**(1):328-357

[17] Parker HM et al. Omega-3 supplementation and non-alcoholic fatty liver disease: A systematic review and meta-analysis. Journal of Hepatology. 2012;**56**(4):944-951

[18] Lee CH et al. Effects of Omega-3 polyunsaturated fatty acid supplementation on non-alcoholic fatty liver: A systematic review and meta-analysis. Nutrients. 2020;**12**(9):2769

[19] Mäkelä TNK et al. Associations of serum n-3 and n-6 polyunsaturated fatty acids with prevalence and incidence of non-alcoholic fatty liver disease. The American Journal of Clinical Nutrition. June 1, 2022:1-12

[20] Dentin R et al. Polyunsaturated fatty acids suppress glycolytic and lipogenic genes through the inhibition of ChREBP nuclear protein translocation. The Journal of Clinical Investigation. 2005;**115**(10):2843-2854

[21] Siriwardhana N, Kalupahana NS, Moustaid-Moussa N. Health benefits of n-3 polyunsaturated fatty acids: Eicosapentaenoic acid and docosahexaenoic acid. Advances in Food and Nutrition Research. 2012;**65**:211-222

[22] Li J et al. The role of vitamins in the pathogenesis of non-alcoholic fatty liver disease. Integrative Medicine Insights. 2016;**11**:19-25

[23] Raza S et al. Vitamins and non-alcoholic fatty liver disease: A molecular insight(★). Liver Research. 2021;**5**(2):62-71

[24] Abe RAM et al. The role of vitamins in non-alcoholic fatty liver disease: A systematic review. Cureus. 2021;**13**(8):e16855

[25] Miller ER 3rd et al. Meta-analysis: High-dosage vitamin E supplementation may increase all-cause mortality. Annals of Internal Medicine. 2005;**142**(1):37-46

[26] Burns J et al. Plant foods and herbal sources of resveratrol. Journal of Agricultural and Food Chemistry. 2002;**50**(11):3337-3340

[27] Elgebaly A et al. Resveratrol supplementation in patients with non-alcoholic fatty liver disease: Systematic review and meta-analysis. Journal of Gastrointestinal and Liver Diseases. 2017;**26**(1):59-67

[28] Andrade JM et al. Resveratrol attenuates hepatic steatosis in high-fat fed mice by decreasing lipogenesis and inflammation. Nutrition. 2014;**30**(7-8):915-919

[29] Faghihzadeh F et al. Resveratrol supplementation improves inflammatory biomarkers in patients with nonalcoholic fatty liver disease. Nutrition Research. 2014;**34**(10):837-843

[30] Leoni S et al. Current guidelines for the management of non-alcoholic fatty liver disease: A systematic review with comparative analysis. World Journal of Gastroenterology. 2018;**24**(30):3361-3373

[31] Anushiravani A et al. Treatment options for nonalcoholic fatty liver disease: A double-blinded randomized placebo-controlled trial. European Journal of Gastroenterology & Hepatology. 2019;**31**(5):613-617

[32] Feng W et al. Randomized trial comparing the effects of gliclazide, liraglutide, and metformin on diabetes with non-alcoholic fatty liver disease. Journal of Diabetes. 2017;**9**(8):800-809

[33] Feng WH et al. Effects of liraglutide, metformin and gliclazide on body composition in patients with both type 2 diabetes and non-alcoholic fatty liver

disease: A randomized trial. Journal of Diabetes Investing. 2019;**10**(2):399-407

[34] Garinis GA et al. Metformin versus dietary treatment in nonalcoholic hepatic steatosis: A randomized study. International Journal of Obesity. 2010;**34**(8):1255-1264

[35] Handzlik G et al. Evaluation of metformin therapy using controlled attenuation parameter and transient elastography in patients with non-alcoholic fatty liver disease. Pharmacological Reports. 2019;**71**(2):183-188

[36] Haukeland JW et al. Metformin in patients with non-alcoholic fatty liver disease: A randomized, controlled trial. Scandinavian Journal of Gastroenterology. 2009;**44**(7):853-860

[37] Idilman R et al. Clinical trial: Insulin-sensitizing agents may reduce consequences of insulin resistance in individuals with non-alcoholic steatohepatitis. Alimentary Pharmacology & Therapeutics. 2008;**28**(2):200-208

[38] Komorizono Y et al. Metformin dose increase versus added linagliptin in non-alcoholic fatty liver disease and type 2 diabetes: An analysis of the J-LINK study. Diabetes, Obesity & Metabolism. 2021;**23**(3):832-837

[39] Nadeau KJ et al. Treatment of non-alcoholic fatty liver disease with metformin versus lifestyle intervention in insulin-resistant adolescents. Pediatric Diabetes. 2009;**10**(1):5-13

[40] Bugianesi E et al. A randomized controlled trial of metformin versus vitamin E or prescriptive diet in nonalcoholic fatty liver disease. The American Journal of Gastroenterology. 2005;**100**(5):1082-1090

[41] Lavine JE et al. Effect of vitamin E or metformin for treatment of nonalcoholic fatty liver disease in children and adolescents: The TONIC randomized controlled trial. JAMA. 2011;**305**(16):1659-1668

[42] Gawrieh S et al. Relationship of enhanced liver fibrosis score with pediatric nonalcoholic fatty liver disease histology and response to vitamin E or metformin. The Journal of Pediatrics. 2021;**239**:161-167.e5

[43] Kinoshita T et al. Comparison of the effects of three kinds of glucose-lowering drugs on non-alcoholic fatty liver disease in patients with type 2 diabetes: A randomized, open-label, three-arm, active control study. Journal of Diabetes Investing. 2020;**11**(6):1612-1622

[44] Yan H et al. Gender differences in the efficacy of pioglitazone treatment in nonalcoholic fatty liver disease patients with abnormal glucose metabolism. Biology of Sex Differences. 2021;**12**(1):1

[45] Yoneda M et al. Comparing the effects of tofogliflozin and pioglitazone in non-alcoholic fatty liver disease patients with type 2 diabetes mellitus (ToPiND study): A randomized prospective open-label controlled trial. BMJ Open Diabetes Research & Care. 2021;**9**(1):e001990

[46] Della Pepa G et al. Pioglitazone even at low dosage improves NAFLD in type 2 diabetes: Clinical and pathophysiological insights from a subgroup of the TOSCA. IT randomised trial. Diabetes Research and Clinical Practice. 2021;**178**:108984

[47] Gastaldelli A et al. PPAR-γ-induced changes in visceral fat and adiponectin levels are associated with improvement of steatohepatitis in patients with NASH. Liver International. 2021;**41**(11):2659-2670

[48] Syed-Abdul MM et al. Fatty acid synthase inhibitor TVB-2640 reduces hepatic de novo lipogenesis in males with metabolic abnormalities. Hepatology. 2020;**72**(1):103-118

[49] Ito D et al. Comparison of Ipragliflozin and pioglitazone effects on nonalcoholic fatty liver disease in patients with type 2 diabetes: A randomized, 24-week, open-label, Active-Controlled Trial. Diabetes Care. 2017;**40**(10):1364-1372

[50] Portillo-Sanchez P et al. Effect of pioglitazone on bone mineral density in patients with nonalcoholic steatohepatitis: A 36-month clinical trial. Journal of Diabetes. 2019;**11**(3):223-231

[51] Cusi K et al. Long-term pioglitazone treatment for patients with nonalcoholic steatohepatitis and prediabetes or type 2 diabetes mellitus: A randomized trial. Annals of Internal Medicine. 2016;**165**(5):305-315

[52] Torres DM et al. Rosiglitazone versus rosiglitazone and metformin versus rosiglitazone and losartan in the treatment of nonalcoholic steatohepatitis in humans: A 12-month randomized, prospective, open- label trial. Hepatology. 2011;**54**(5):1631-1639

[53] Armstrong MJ et al. Glucagon-like peptide 1 decreases lipotoxicity in non-alcoholic steatohepatitis. Journal of Hepatology. 2016;**64**(2):399-408

[54] Bouchi R et al. Reduction of visceral fat by liraglutide is associated with ameliorations of hepatic steatosis, albuminuria, and micro-inflammation in type 2 diabetic patients with insulin treatment: A randomized control trial. Endocrine Journal. 2017;**64**(3):269-281

[55] Fan H et al. Exenatide improves type 2 diabetes concomitant with non-alcoholic fatty liver disease. Arquivos Brasileiros de Endocrinologia e Metabologia. 2013;**57**(9):702-708

[56] Guo W et al. Liraglutide or insulin glargine treatments improves hepatic fat in obese patients with type 2 diabetes and nonalcoholic fatty liver disease in twenty-six weeks: A randomized placebo-controlled trial. Diabetes Research and Clinical Practice. 2020;**170**:108487

[57] Hartman ML et al. Effects of novel dual GIP and GLP-1 receptor agonist Tirzepatide on biomarkers of nonalcoholic steatohepatitis in patients with type 2 diabetes. Diabetes Care. 2020;**43**(6):1352-1355

[58] Khoo J et al. Comparative effects of liraglutide 3 mg vs structured lifestyle modification on body weight, liver fat and liver function in obese patients with non-alcoholic fatty liver disease: A pilot randomized trial. Diabetes, Obesity & Metabolism. 2017;**19**(12):1814-1817

[59] Khoo J et al. Randomized trial comparing effects of weight loss by liraglutide with lifestyle modification in non-alcoholic fatty liver disease. Liver International. 2019;**39**(5):941-949

[60] Kuchay MS et al. Effect of dulaglutide on liver fat in patients with type 2 diabetes and NAFLD: Randomised controlled trial (D-LIFT trial). Diabetologia. 2020;**63**(11):2434-2445

[61] Smits MM et al. Twelve week liraglutide or sitagliptin does not affect hepatic fat in type 2 diabetes: A randomised placebo-controlled trial. Diabetologia. 2016;**59**(12):2588-2593

[62] Yan J et al. Liraglutide, Sitagliptin, and insulin glargine added to metformin: The effect on body weight and intrahepatic lipid in patients with type 2 diabetes mellitus and nonalcoholic

fatty liver disease. Hepatology. 2019;**69**(6):2414-2426

[63] Zhang LY et al. Effect of liraglutide therapy on serum fetuin a in patients with type 2 diabetes and non-alcoholic fatty liver disease. Clinics and Research in Hepatology and Gastroenterology. 2020;**44**(5):674-680

[64] Eriksson JW et al. Effects of dapagliflozin and n-3 carboxylic acids on non-alcoholic fatty liver disease in people with type 2 diabetes: A double-blind randomised placebo-controlled study. Diabetologia. 2018;**61**(9):1923-1934

[65] Shibuya T et al. Luseogliflozin improves liver fat deposition compared to metformin in type 2 diabetes patients with non-alcoholic fatty liver disease: A prospective randomized controlled pilot study. Diabetes, Obesity & Metabolism. 2018;**20**(2):438-442

[66] Qiang S et al. Treatment with the SGLT2 inhibitor luseogliflozin improves nonalcoholic steatohepatitis in a rodent model with diabetes mellitus. Diabetology and Metabolic Syndrome. 2015;7:104

[67] Kuchay MS et al. Effect of Empagliflozin on liver fat in patients with type 2 diabetes and nonalcoholic fatty liver disease: A randomized controlled trial (E-LIFT trial). Diabetes Care. 2018;**41**(8):1801-1808

[68] Athyros VG et al. The use of statins alone, or in combination with pioglitazone and other drugs, for the treatment of non-alcoholic fatty liver disease/non-alcoholic steatohepatitis and related cardiovascular risk. An Expert Panel Statement. Metabolism. 2017;**71**:17-32

[69] Athyros VG et al. Statins: An under-appreciated asset for the prevention and the treatment of NAFLD or NASH and the related cardiovascular risk. Current Vascular Pharmacology. 2018;**16**(3):246-253

[70] Torres-Peña JD, Martín-Piedra L, Fuentes-Jiménez F. Statins in non-alcoholic steatohepatitis. Frontiers in Cardiovascular Medicine. 2021;**8**:777131

[71] Eslami L et al. Statins for non-alcoholic fatty liver disease and non-alcoholic steatohepatitis. Cochrane Database of Systematic Reviews. 2013;**12**:Cd008623

[72] Cho Y et al. Ezetimibe combination therapy with statin for non-alcoholic fatty liver disease: An open-label randomized controlled trial (ESSENTIAL study). BMC Medicine. 2022;**20**(1):93

[73] Loomba R et al. Ezetimibe for the treatment of nonalcoholic steatohepatitis: Assessment by novel magnetic resonance imaging and magnetic resonance elastography in a randomized trial (MOZART trial). Hepatology. 2015;**61**(4):1239-1250

[74] Lucas C et al. A systematic review of the present and future of non-alcoholic fatty liver disease. Clinical and Experimental Hepatology. 2018;**4**(3):165-174

[75] Loomba R et al. GS-0976 reduces hepatic steatosis and fibrosis markers in patients with nonalcoholic fatty liver disease. Gastroenterology. 2018;**155**(5):1463-1473.e6

[76] Amin NB et al. Efficacy and safety of an orally administered DGAT2 inhibitor alone or coadministered with a liver-targeted ACC inhibitor in adults with non-alcoholic steatohepatitis (NASH): Rationale and design of the phase II, dose-ranging, dose-finding,

randomised, placebo-controlled MIRNA (metabolic interventions to resolve NASH with fibrosis) study. BMJ Open. 2022;**12**(3):e056159

[77] Calle RA et al. ACC inhibitor alone or co-administered with a DGAT2 inhibitor in patients with non-alcoholic fatty liver disease: Two parallel, placebo-controlled, randomized phase 2a trials. Nature Medicine. 2021;**27**(10):1836-1848

[78] Stiede K et al. Acetyl-coenzyme a carboxylase inhibition reduces de novo lipogenesis in overweight male subjects: A randomized, double-blind, crossover study. Hepatology. 2017;**66**(2):324-334

[79] Matsumoto M et al. Acetyl-CoA carboxylase 1 and 2 inhibition ameliorates steatosis and hepatic fibrosis in a MC4R knockout murine model of nonalcoholic steatohepatitis. PLoS One. 2020;**15**(1):e0228212

[80] Goedeke L et al. Acetyl-CoA carboxylase inhibition reverses NAFLD and hepatic insulin resistance but promotes hypertriglyceridemia in rodents. Hepatology. 2018;**68**(6):2197-2211

[81] Tamura YO et al. Selective acetyl-CoA carboxylase 1 inhibitor improves hepatic steatosis and hepatic fibrosis in a preclinical nonalcoholic steatohepatitis model. The Journal of Pharmacology and Experimental Therapeutics. 2021;**379**(3):280-289

[82] Neokosmidis G, Cholongitas E, Tziomalos K. Acetyl-CoA carboxylase inhibitors in non-alcoholic steatohepatitis: Is there a benefit? World Journal of Gastroenterology. 2021;**27**(39):6522-6526

[83] Beysen C et al. Inhibition of fatty acid synthase with FT-4101 safely reduces hepatic de novo lipogenesis and steatosis in obese subjects with non-alcoholic fatty liver disease: Results from two early-phase randomized trials. Diabetes, Obesity & Metabolism. 2021;**23**(3):700-710

[84] Loomba R et al. TVB-2640 (FASN inhibitor) for the treatment of nonalcoholic steatohepatitis: FASCINATE-1, a randomized, placebo-controlled phase 2a trial. Gastroenterology. 2021;**161**(5):1475-1486

[85] Wiest R et al. Targeting the gut-liver axis in liver disease. Journal of Hepatology. 2017;**67**(5):1084-1103

[86] Okour M, Brigandi RA, Tenero D. A population analysis of the DGAT1 inhibitor GSK3008356 and its effect on endogenous and meal-induced triglyceride turnover in healthy subjects. Fundamental & Clinical Pharmacology. 2019;**33**(5):567-580

[87] Amin NB et al. Targeting diacylglycerol acyltransferase 2 for the treatment of nonalcoholic steatohepatitis. Science Translational Medicine. 2019;**11**(520):eaav9701

[88] Loomba R et al. Novel antisense inhibition of diacylglycerol O-acyltransferase 2 for treatment of non-alcoholic fatty liver disease: A multicentre, double-blind, randomised, placebo-controlled phase 2 trial. The Lancet Gastroenterology & Hepatology. 2020;**5**(9):829-838

[89] Younossi ZM et al. Obeticholic acid impact on quality of life in patients with nonalcoholic steatohepatitis: REGENERATE 18-month interim analysis. Clinical Gastroenterology and Hepatology. Jul 15, 2021:S1542-3565

[90] Rinella ME et al. Non-invasive evaluation of response to obeticholic acid in patients with NASH: Results from

the REGENERATE study. Journal of Hepatology. 2022;**76**(3):536-548

[91] Hameed B et al. Clinical and metabolic effects associated with weight changes and obeticholic acid in non-alcoholic steatohepatitis. Alimentary Pharmacology & Therapeutics. 2018;**47**(5):645-656

[92] Mudaliar S et al. Efficacy and safety of the farnesoid X receptor agonist obeticholic acid in patients with type 2 diabetes and nonalcoholic fatty liver disease. Gastroenterology. 2013;**145**(3):574-82.e1

[93] Neuschwander-Tetri BA et al. Farnesoid X nuclear receptor ligand obeticholic acid for non-cirrhotic, non-alcoholic steatohepatitis (FLINT): A multicentre, randomised, placebo-controlled trial. Lancet. 2015;**385**(9972):956-965

[94] Pockros PJ et al. CONTROL: A randomized phase 2 study of obeticholic acid and atorvastatin on lipoproteins in nonalcoholic steatohepatitis patients. Liver International. 2019;**39**(11):2082-2093

[95] Ratziu V et al. REGENERATE: Design of a pivotal, randomised, phase 3 study evaluating the safety and efficacy of obeticholic acid in patients with fibrosis due to nonalcoholic steatohepatitis. Contemporary Clinical Trials. 2019;**84**:105803

[96] Siddiqui MS et al. Impact of obeticholic acid on the lipoprotein profile in patients with non-alcoholic steatohepatitis. Journal of Hepatology. 2020;**72**(1):25-33

[97] Younossi ZM et al. Obeticholic acid for the treatment of non-alcoholic steatohepatitis: Interim analysis from a multicentre, randomised, placebo-controlled phase 3 trial. Lancet. 2019;**394**(10215):2184-2196

[98] Alam S et al. Effect of telmisartan on histological activity and fibrosis of non-alcoholic steatohepatitis: A 1-year randomized control trial. Saudi Journal of Gastroenterology. 2016;**22**(1):69-76

[99] McPherson S et al. A randomised controlled trial of losartan as an anti-fibrotic agent in non-alcoholic steatohepatitis. PLoS One. 2017;**12**(4):e0175717

[100] Wasta Esmail VA, Al-Nimer MSM, Mohammed MO. Effects of orlistat or Telmisartan on the serum free fatty acids in non-alcoholic fatty liver disease patients: An open-labeled randomized controlled study. The Turkish Journal of Gastroenterology. 2022;**33**(5):421-426

[101] Pydyn N et al. New therapeutic strategies in nonalcoholic fatty liver disease: A focus on promising drugs for nonalcoholic steatohepatitis. Pharmacological Reports. 2020;**72**(1):1-12

[102] Ferguson D, Finck BN. Emerging therapeutic approaches for the treatment of NAFLD and type 2 diabetes mellitus. Nature Reviews. Endocrinology. 2021;**17**(8):484-495

[103] Makri E, Goulas A, Polyzos SA. Epidemiology, pathogenesis, diagnosis and emerging treatment of nonalcoholic fatty liver disease. Archives of Medical Research. 2021;**52**(1):25-37

[104] Fernández T et al. Lifestyle changes in patients with non-alcoholic fatty liver disease: A systematic review and meta-analysis. PLoS One. 2022;**17**(2):e0263931

[105] Petersen KF et al. Reversal of nonalcoholic hepatic steatosis, hepatic insulin resistance, and hyperglycemia

by moderate weight reduction in patients with type 2 diabetes. Diabetes. 2005;**54**(3):603-608

[106] Kleiner DE et al. Design and validation of a histological scoring system for nonalcoholic fatty liver disease. Hepatology. 2005;**41**(6):1313-1321

[107] Katsagoni CN et al. Improvements in clinical characteristics of patients with non-alcoholic fatty liver disease, after an intervention based on the Mediterranean lifestyle: A randomised controlled clinical trial. The British Journal of Nutrition. 2018;**120**(2):164-175

[108] Yaskolka Meir A et al. Effect of green-Mediterranean diet on intrahepatic fat: The DIRECT PLUS randomised controlled trial. Gut. 2021;**70**(11):2085-2095

[109] George ES et al. Impact of a Mediterranean diet on hepatic and metabolic outcomes in non-alcoholic fatty liver disease: The MEDINA randomised controlled trial. Liver International. 2022;**42**(6):1308-1322

[110] Jimenez LS et al. Impact of weight regain on the evolution of non-alcoholic fatty liver disease after roux-en-Y gastric bypass: A 3-year follow-up. Obesity Surgery. 2018;**28**(10):3131-3135

[111] Marin-Alejandre BA et al. Effects of two personalized dietary strategies during a 2-year intervention in subjects with nonalcoholic fatty liver disease: A randomized trial. Liver International. 2021;**41**(7):1532-1544

[112] Gjesing AP et al. Fasting and oral glucose-stimulated levels of glucose-dependent insulinotropic polypeptide (GIP) and glucagon-like peptide-1 (GLP-1) are highly familial traits. Diabetologia. 2012;**55**(5):1338-1345

[113] Montemayor S et al. Effect of dietary and lifestyle interventions on the amelioration of NAFLD in patients with metabolic syndrome: The FLIPAN study. Nutrients. 2022;**14**(11):2223

[114] Noto D et al. Lifestyle versus ezetimibe plus lifestyle in patients with biopsy-proven non-alcoholic steatohepatitis (LISTEN): A double-blind randomised placebo-controlled trial. Nutrition, Metabolism, and Cardiovascular Diseases. 2022;**32**(5):1288-1291

[115] Mascaró CM et al. Effect of a six-month lifestyle intervention on the physical activity and fitness status of adults with NAFLD and metabolic syndrome. Nutrients. 2022;**14**(9):1813

[116] Kenđel Jovanović G et al. Metabolic and hepatic effects of energy-reduced anti-inflammatory diet in younger adults with obesity. Canadian Journal of Gastroenterology & Hepatology. 2021;**2021**:6649142

[117] Franco I et al. Physical activity and low glycemic index Mediterranean diet: Main and modification effects on NAFLD score. Results from a randomized clinical trial. Nutrients. 2020;**13**(1):66

[118] Ristic-Medic D et al. Calorie-restricted Mediterranean and low-fat diets affect fatty acid status in individuals with nonalcoholic fatty liver disease. Nutrients. 2020;**13**(1):15

[119] Evert AB, Franz MJ. Why weight loss maintenance is difficult. Diabetes Spectrum: A Publication of the American Diabetes Association. 2017;**30**(3):153-156

[120] Lonardo A, Arab JP, Arrese M. Perspectives on precision medicine approaches to NAFLD diagnosis and management. Advances in Therapy. 2021;**38**(5):2130-2158

[121] Hallsworth K, Avery L, Trenell MI. Targeting lifestyle behavior change in adults with NAFLD during a 20-min consultation: Summary of the dietary and exercise literature. Current Gastroenterology Reports. 2016;**18**(3):11

[122] Borek AJ et al. Group-based diet and physical activity weight-loss interventions: A systematic review and meta-analysis of randomised controlled trials. Applied Psychology. Health and Well-Being. 2018;**10**(1):62-86

[123] Caussy C, Aubin A, Loomba R. The relationship between type 2 diabetes, NAFLD, and cardiovascular risk. Current Diabetes Reports. 2021;**21**(5):15

Chapter 6

Necessity of Herbal Medicine in the Management of Metabolic Syndrome

Sarvesh Sabarathinam, Rajappan Chandra Satish Kumar and Thangavel Mahalingam Vijayakumar

Abstract

People are more susceptible to a variety of diseases based on their lifestyle and occupational patterns. Metabolic syndrome (MS) is a worldwide health issue that is linked to a variety of risk factors, including hyperglycemia, dyslipidemia, hypertension, and obesity. Herbal medicine has been used for a long time. Herbal medicines have emerged as a significant source and major focus for future drug development and human health care. Botanicals may be useful for treating or preventing metabolic syndrome because they often have a wide range of biologically active compounds that can work together to boost each other's effectiveness or have a synergistic effect, giving more benefit than a single chemical substance. Some extracts of botanicals frequently contain natural active components that act on multiple biological targets, creating an opportunity to concurrently resolve multiple defects associated with metabolic syndrome. To find out if botanicals can be used to treat metabolic syndrome as a group, trials must be stratified to look at differences in disease severity, age, gender, and genetic variation in the sample populations.

Keywords: lifestyle disease, metabolic syndrome, diabetes, obesity, herbal medicines

1. Introduction

Lifestyle diseases are distinguished as changes in the metabolism profile of a population and are directly proportional to their day-to-day habits. The primary factors that induce lifestyle diseases include unorganized food habits, uninhabited exercise activities, etc. Metabolic syndrome is a common metabolic condition that is being exacerbated by rising obesity rates. The metabolic syndrome, also known as syndrome X, insulin resistance, and other terms, is a pathologic condition characterized by abdominal obesity, insulin resistance, hypertension, and hyperlipidemia, according to the World Health Organization. Prothrombotic conditions, proinflammatory states, nonalcoholic fatty liver disease, and reproductive abnormalities are some of the other comorbidities [1]. Diabetes is a chronic metabolic disorder and it puts tremendous pressure on patients as well as their socioeconomic status. In recent decades, the prevalence of diabetes has been raised gradually in certain developed countries.

As per the International Diabetes Federation (IDF) data, the diabetes prevalence may increase by 693 million in the year 2045 if successful measures of treatment are not implemented [1]. Incidence and prevalence rates of diabetes in Indian populations are illustrated in **Figure 1**.

The incidence of diabetes has risen significantly in recent decades, and it is expected to be higher in the upcoming decades. These specific complaints, in addition to cardiovascular complications, respiratory disorders, and cancers, are directly responsible for 80% of all premature noncommunicable disease (NCD) deaths [2].

Data from IDF show that diabetes is a rising concern in India. The estimated rate of diabetes patients is 8.7%, and the age range is between 20 and 70 years [3]. Formal paraphrase diabetes mellitus is a metabolic disorder correlated with carbohydrate, fat, and protein metabolism and is followed by insulin deficiency and/or insulin resistance. Diabetes mellitus has the following characteristic signs and symptoms: thirst, polyuria, blurring of vision, and weight loss [4]. The metabolic syndrome

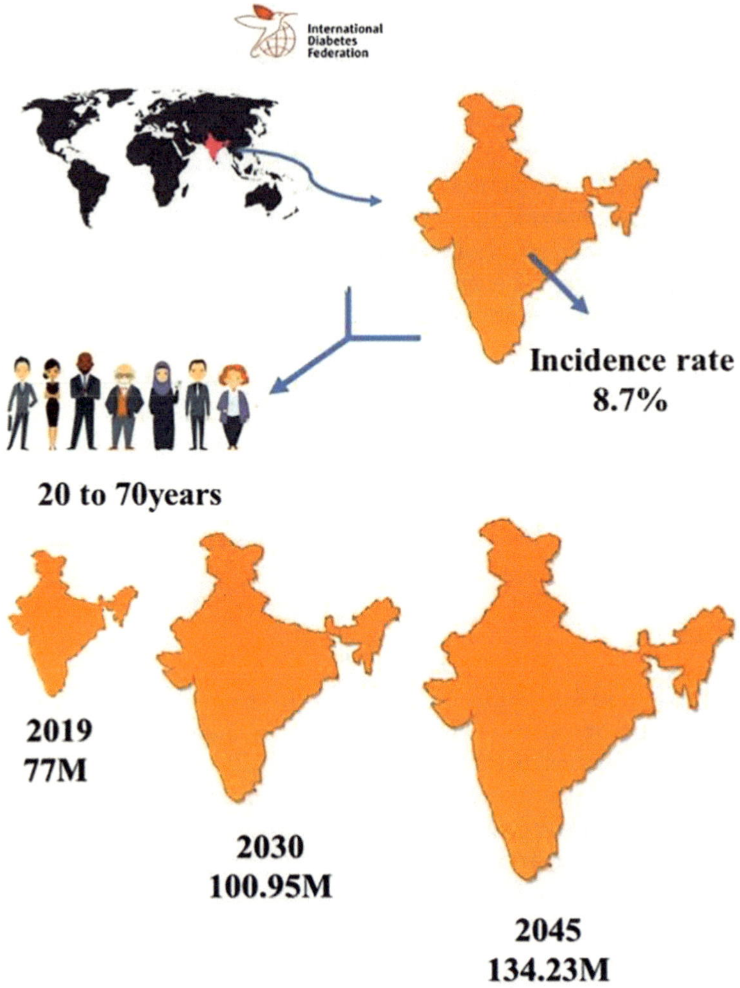

Figure 1.
Incidence rate of diabetes in India in millions.

has been around for over 80 years. Over the last two decades, the number of people with metabolic syndrome has risen dramatically worldwide. This rise is linked to the worldwide obesity and diabetes epidemic. The metabolic syndrome increases the risk of diabetes and cardiovascular disease, necessitating the development of measures to combat the oncoming global epidemic [5].

According to studies published in the previous decade, approximately one-quarter to one-third of adults from various ethnic origins meet metabolic syndrome requirements. Metabolic syndrome becomes more common as people get older [6]. Type 2 diabetes mellitus (T2DM) was shown to be more common in specific ethnic groups, with 15% of American Indians having T2DM and only 4.30% of Chinese Americans having T2DM. South Asian Americans have a greater frequency of metabolic syndrome and abdominal obesity than other ethnic groups [7]. The factor that increases the risk of the development of the metabolic disorder is positive family history smoking, Increasing age, obesity, low socioeconomic status, Mexican-American ethnicity, postmenopausal status, physical inactivity, sugary drinks and soft drink consumption, excessive alcohol consumption, Western dietary patterns, low cardiorespiratory fitness, excessive television watching, use of antiretroviral drugs in human immunodeficiency virus (HIV) infection, atypical antipsychotic drug use (e.g., clozapine) [8]. Insulin resistance and hyperinsulinemia are regarded as key risk factors for the development of metabolic syndrome, and they may also play a role in the pathophysiology of its metabolic components [9]. Body fat distribution, particularly visceral fat accumulation, is a significant predictor of the metabolic syndrome, a collection of diabetogenic, atherogenic, prothrombotic, and proinflammatory metabolic abnormalities marked by dysfunctional adipocytes and dysregulated adipocytokine production (hypoadiponectinemia) [10]. The "lipid triad" of high plasma triglycerides, low levels of high-density lipoprotein cholesterol (HDL-C), and a preponderance of small, dense low-density lipoprotein (LDL) particles are the main components of the dyslipidemia of the metabolic syndrome, which most likely causes atherosclerotic cardiovascular disease. Therapeutic lifestyle changes are a cornerstone of treatment. Drug therapy may be indicated if it does not treat dyslipidemia. The first-line treatment for reducing LDL-C is with statins [11]. In patients with metabolic syndrome, visceral fat reduction combined with lifestyle changes might be a beneficial therapy for preventing atherosclerotic cardiovascular disease (ACVD) [10].

2. Overview of complementary and alternative medicines (CAM)

CAM is a group of therapeutic and diagnostic principles that are often practiced by patients along with conventional therapies. CAM is normally not appreciated by the majority of the medical profession as traditional or mainstream medical approaches. Integrative medicine is an approach to medical care that combines standard medicine with CAM practices that are shown to be effective and safe [3].

CAM therapies are widely used all over the world. Since the majority of patients are not satisfied with their existing treatment pattern, patients do believe alternative therapies are suitable for their illnesses since they are natural and free from toxicity. Herbal medicine is the preparation of biologically active natural products that have therapeutic value. The use of herbal medicines in developed countries has expanded in the latter half of the twentieth century. Recently, the WHO estimated that 80% of people rely on herbal medicines for some aspect of their primary health care needs. More than 70% of the Indian population still uses these plant-based medicinal products for their needs. As a significance of dissatisfaction with conventional medicine, herbal remedies are becoming increasingly popular in developed nations. Herbal remedies are widely thought to be innately safe because they are "natural." Their effects are generally related to the pharmacological features and dose levels of their active ingredient, rather than their natural origin. Herbal medicines, on the other hand, can be toxic if used inappropriately or as a substitute for conventional medications. Toxic effects can indeed be linked to a variety of pharmaceutical reasons, such as ingredient toxicity, preparation contamination by pesticides, microbes, heavy metals, or synthetic pharmaceuticals. As a result, before using any herbal medicine, both users and doctors and practitioners should be capable of making the greatest risk-benefit assessment possible [12].

For the treatment of diabetes and its consequences, several different plants have been employed individually or in formulations. The active ingredients in this herbal mixture are not well described, which is one of the primary flaws. It's critical to understand the active ingredients and their molecular interactions, as this will aid in determining the product's medicinal efficacy and standardizing the manufacturing process. The absence of scientific and clinical data showing herbal medicine's efficacy and safety is a major impediment to its incorporation into modern medical procedures. Clinical research on herbal medications is required, as are the development of simple bioassays for biological standardization, pharmacological and toxicological evaluation, and the development of numerous animal models for toxicity and safety testing. Widely practiced alternative therapies in the management of metabolic syndromes are herbal supplements, acupuncture therapy, massage therapy, meditation, and yoga therapy. Plant-based medicinal products are highly consumed by the

Study participants	Conclusion	Reference
34 postmenopausal women aged 50–70 years were randomly assigned to exercise and placebo	The use of isoflavones when body weight remains stable seems to enhance the beneficial effects of mixed-exercise training on body composition and CRP in overweight or obese postmenopausal women.	[4]
A randomized, double-blind placebo-controlled study of a herbal dietary supplement in Overweight men and women of Sixty-seven subjects	This herbal mixture of Ma Huang and Guarana effectively promoted short-term weight and fat loss	[14]
A randomized, double-blind, placebo-controlled clinical trial with 80 obese participants without any disease were recruited randomly into actiponin and placebo groups	Actiponin supplementation may be effective for treating obese individuals	[6]
80 obese women were randomly assigned for either ginger (2-g ginger rhizomes powder per day) or placebo supplements (corn starch with the same amount)	Ginger consumption has potential in managing obesity	[7]
Double-blinded, randomized subjects with BMI ≧27 was randomly divided into control (n = 18) and an oat-treated (n = 16) group	Consumption of oat reduced obesity, abdominal fat, and improved lipid profiles and liver functions	[8]

Table 1.
Clinical evidences of plant-based medicinal products in the management of metabolic syndrome.

majority of the population. **Table 1** discusses the clinical evidence of herbal supplements in the management of obesity.

3. Uses of herbal medicine in the management of metabolic syndrome

Diabetes mellitus (DM): DM is a metabolic condition that affects millions of people worldwide. Diabetes is caused by a shortage of insulin or inadequate insulin synthesis in the pancreas. Even though several synthetic medications have been produced, none of them provides a complete cure. Long-term use of some synthetic compounds creates significant adverse effects, but there is still a desire for nontoxic, low-cost medications. Throughout human history, traditional therapies have been a highly regarded source of medicine. These are widely utilized around the world, demonstrating that herbs are becoming an increasingly important aspect of modern and high-tech medicine. A total of 21,000 plants are utilized for therapeutic reasons around the world, according to the World Health Organization (WHO), and there are around 400 plants available for the treatment of diabetes among them [13]. **Table 2** discusses the frequently used plant-based medicinal products in the management of metabolic syndrome.

Several herbs, comprising extracts or bioactive constituents derived from plants, can be primarily used to treat metabolic syndrome, also in nano-formulated pharmaceutical forms. For this global concern, researchers and physicians are exploring novel, safe, complementary, and alternative therapeutic approaches. Herbal remedies are found to be a promising way to lose weight and body fat. The benefits of herbal medicines such as antihyperglycemic, anti-obesity, anti-inflammatory properties, and antioxidant agents were examined in different preclinical and clinical investigations [15]. The advantages of employing medicinal plants as just a safe, economical, approachable, and organic alternative healthcare solution for the treatment of metabolic diseases' health outcomes.

Herbal medicines promote insulin secretion and cardiovascular health while reducing gluconeogenesis, inflammation, and oxidative stress. To manage diabetes and its consequences, various plant extracts have been proposed. Nanostructured formulations of herbal extracts can improve their anti-diabetic effects by regulating their pharmacokinetics and making them more available to the body [16].

Name of the plant-based medicinal products	Therapeutic effect
Fennel	Aids in the reduction of fat and sugar absorption
Cinnamon	↓Low-density lipoprotein and triglycerides
Gimena	Inhibits the absorption of glucose and the buildup of fatty acids.
Aloe vera	Enhance carbohydrate metabolism and minimizes glucose intolerance caused by obesity
Moringa	Triglycerides and elevated blood glucose reduction
Bitter melon and fenugreek	Increases insulin sensitivity, reduce low-density lipoprotein and Triglycerides

Table 2.
Few plant-based medicinal products in the management of metabolic syndrome.

Considering long-term use of some synthetic compounds creates significant adverse effects, there is still a necessity for nontoxic, low-cost medications. Throughout the history of mankind, traditional therapies have been a highly regarded source of treatment. These are usually employed around the world, demonstrating that herbs are becoming an increasingly important aspect of modern and high-tech medicine. The low level of side effects associated with herbal pharmaceuticals is one of their key advantages, and this has encouraged several researchers to develop novel molecules for the treatment of diabetes. Recent breakthroughs in the field of herbal medications to treat diabetes, prevent diabetes-related secondary problems, and numerous herbal compounds in various stages of clinical trials [13].

Various herbal medicines such as capsicum annum of the capsicum family showed anti-diabetic effects by increasing insulin sensitivity in peripheral tissues, improvement in glucose tolerance, protection of β cells from apoptosis, and reduction of insulin level in clinical studies. Capsaicin (the active ingredient in the capsicum family) stimulates GLP-1 secretion, thus increasing glucagon level in the blood and thus decreasing Ghrelin level (orexigenic hormone). There is evidence of inhibition of α-amylase and α-glucosidase activity via preclinical studies [17].

Saffron, a dried stigma of Crocus sativus used as a spice with coloring properties, demonstrated an anti-hyperglycemic effect by reducing the serum blood glucose level in streptozotocin-induced diabetic rats and showed an antioxidant effect. It also reverses the pancreatic damage, phosphorylation of AMP-activated protein kinase and mitogen-activated protein kinase (which play an important role in glucose uptake and insulin sensitivity) [18].

As per recent studies, the most potent plants for fasting blood glucose (FBS) are green tea (at 150 and 1000 mg/day), *Hibiscus sabdariffa* (at 1000 mg/day), tea (at a dose of 10 g/day), cinnamon (at doses of 550 and 3000 mg/day), and many more. A remarkable reduction in HbA1C was also noted by taking *Hibiscus sabdariffa*, *Citrus aurantium*, Sea buckthorn, Bilberries, a combination of *Proteus vulgaris* and *Ceratonia siliqua*, and a combination of grape seeds and pine bark. Moreover, it has been established in two studies that two plants, chia and *Rhus coriaria* L., can boost insulin secretion [15].

After months of consumption, *Aloe vera* extract capsules (300 mg/kg) lowered fasting blood glucose, TG, LDL, and HbA1c levels. For 3 months, *Aloe vera* powder (100, 200 mg/kg) was administered to reduce fasting and postprandial glucose, blood pressure, and HDL levels [19].

Other herbal medicines or extracts such as bitter melon, mostly used by the Asian population, reduce Fasting Blood Sugar (FBS) and post-prandial blood sugar (PPBS) by acting on the GLUT-4 receptor. Fenugreek improved blood glucose levels and increased insulin sensitivity when combined with anti-diabetic therapy. Yuquan Wan, a Chinese extract administered for 1 month, decreased FBS and improved diabetic-related complications. Xioake Wan (XAX), a Chinese medicine, showcased a significant improvement in blood lipid and blood glucose parameters when combined with anti-diabetic drugs and enhanced insulin sensitivity [20]. Most people's hypertension goes untreated or uncontrolled. The availability, cost, and side effects of antihypertensive medicines hinder the effective treatment of hypertension. Conventional treatment was unable to alleviate several hypertension-related symptoms [21]. Lifestyle adjustments, dietary changes, and the use of combination therapy with herbs are some of the most commonly used alternative measures for decreasing high blood pressure. Herbal medicines, in general, have no negative side effects while also providing additional benefits. Herbal remedies are available in almost all health stores and can be purchased without the need for a prescription. Some herbs can even be cultivated in your backyard. These treatments are ideal for people who are allergic to a variety of medications.

The leading cause of sickness worldwide is hypertension. Patients who are prescribed pharmacological therapy may refuse it due to the asymptomatic nature of their hypertension, opting for other remedies instead. Herbal medicines such as DiaNo decoction, Yiqi Huaju Recipe, Daotan decoction, Gegen Shanzha decoction, Qinggan Jiangtang tablet, Modified Banxia Baizhu Tianma decoction, Pinggan Jiangya pill, Huanglian Wendan decoction, Xueguan Ruanhua decoction, Shengjiangtongmai powder, and Shenling Jianpihuashi decoction showed a significant reduction in blood pressure in many clinical studies. It was also found that Shenling Jianpihuashi decoction had the same effect as nifedipine in animal studies, and a double-blind study, saffron, and its constituents exhibit vasomodulatory effects and improve endothelium-dependent acetylcholine (ACh) relaxation via the endothelial nitric oxide pathway. Various animal-based studies and a double-blind study showed decreased systolic blood pressure. It also showed an effect via blocking calcium release in the cytosol [18]. In preclinical studies, Panax Ginseng (3 g/kg) used for 12 weeks reduced arterial stiffness and systolic blood pressure via endothelial nitric oxide synthase (eNOS) activation and the nitric oxide pathway [22]. Several of the synthetic medications employed possess unfavorable side effects. Herbal supplements can be used in addition to or instead of pharmaceutical treatments for weight loss and maintenance. They are beneficial, safer, and much less expensive than pharmaceutical drugs. Medicinal herbs include pharmacodynamic bioactive chemicals that have a synergistic and additive medicinal impact on the treatment of metabolic diseases. Herbs possess anti-obesity effects through a variety of mechanisms, including appetite suppression and satiety enhancement, increased energy expenditure, low-fat digestion, and increased fat lipolysis [23].

Obesity is a metabolic condition where there is an abnormal accumulation of fat in the body, and it is linked to the augmentation of disorders such as hypertension, dyslipidemia, type 2 diabetes mellitus, osteoarthritis, kidney disease, sleep disorders, etc. There are currently only a few effective medicines for treating obesity, despite ongoing investment in research. As a result, patients and researchers are seeking complementary and alternative treatment options for obesity, such as the use of medicinal plants and their products. According to research findings, herbal plants could be an alternative therapy for hyperlipidemia in patients who are statin-intolerant or unwilling to take modern antihyperlipidemic medicines.

In several clinical studies, herbal plants have been shown to reduce body fat percentage (BF%), fat mass (FM), and fat free mass (FFM) in several ways. FM and BF% were significantly decreased by green tea (green tea at dose of 6000 mg/day and catechins at doses of 458, 468, and 886 mg/day), *H. sabdariffa* (dose of 75 mg/day), *Phaseolus vulgaris* (at dose of 445 mg/day, G. cambogia (at doses of 2400 and 3000 mg/day, *Ecklonia cava* (at doses of 72 and 144 mg/day, cumin (dose of 3000 mg/day, Coleus forskolii (at dose of 250 mg/day), Sorghum tea (at dose of 1000 ml/day), *Gynostemma pentaphyllum* (at dose of 450 mg/day), and cinnamon (at dose of 550 mg/day), *Ginkgo biloba*. L (120 mg/kg) with Metformin (500 mg) in the 90 days of treatment showed a reduction in HbA1c, BMI, and fasting serum glucose level [24].

In a clinical trial using capsaicinoid (6 mg/kg) for 12 weeks, it was found that there was a significant fat reduction. Capsaicin, a water-soluble derivative of homovanillic acid and an active ingredient of capsicum plants, is responsible for various anti-inflammatory properties in skin problems, gastritis problems, migraines, hemorrhoids, anorexia, etc. Recent studies conducted via in vivo and vitro methods demonstrated that capsaicin acts as an antihyperlipidemic agent by activating peroxisome proliferator activated receptor (PPAR-) and by reducing intestinal absorption and elevation of bile acid secretion. Thus, activation of peroxisome proliferator-activated receptors (*PPARs*) leads to a reduction of LDL, triglycerides, and serum cholesterol and an increase of HDL [17].

4. Conclusion

Heart disease, aortic stenosis, atrial fibrillation, stroke, and even thromboembolic illness can all occur in patients with lifestyle diseases. Evidence now suggests that the risk of ischemic stroke in people with metabolic syndrome is significantly higher than previously anticipated. Other issues linked to metabolic syndrome include a higher chance of cancers in the colon, kidney, and gallbladder. In addition, metabolic syndrome may increase the risk of cognitive dysfunction. Finally, patients with metabolic syndrome are more likely to fall into the polypharmacy category, which means they will have higher medical expenses, be more likely to be impoverished, and have difficulty accessing high-quality treatment. Crude drugs are safe and can be expected to have the effects of improving metabolic syndrome. Treatment with complementary and alternative medicine will become effective methods. In this case, to prevent the drugs' induced secondary complications and economic problems, patients believe in alternative therapies such as plant medicinal products since they are safe, reliable, free from toxicity, and cost-effective.

Acknowledgements

We would like to thank all the healthcare professionals.

Funding

No funding has been raised for this study.

Competing interests

The authors declare no competing interests.

Consent to publish

The consent was taken from all coauthors.

Author details

Sarvesh Sabarathinam[1], Rajappan Chandra Satish Kumar[1*]
and Thangavel Mahalingam Vijayakumar[2]

1 Drug Testing Laboratory, Interdisciplinary Institute of Indian System of Medicine (IIISM), SRM Institute of Science and Technology, Kattankulathur, Tamil Nadu, India

2 Department of Pharmacy Practice, SRM College of Pharmacy, SRM Institute of Science and Technology, Kattankulathur, Tamil Nadu, India

*Address all correspondence to: ayursatish@gmail.com

References

[1] Cornier MA et al. The metabolic syndrome (in Eng). Endocrine Reviews. 2008;**29**(7):777-822

[2] Lin X et al. Global, regional, and national burden and trend of diabetes in 195 countries and territories: An analysis from 1990 to 2025. Scientific Reports. 2020;**10**(1):14790

[3] Kaveeshwar SA, Cornwall J. The current state of diabetes mellitus in India (in eng). The Australasian Medical Journal. 2014;**7**(1):45-48

[4] American Diabetes A. Diagnosis and classification of diabetes mellitus (in eng). Diabetes Care. 2009;**32**(Suppl. 1): S62-S67

[5] Khan MAB, Hashim MJ, King JK, Govender RD, Mustafa H, Al Kaabi J. Epidemiology of type 2 diabetes—Global burden of disease and forecasted trends (in eng). Journal of Epidemiology and Global Health. 2020;**10**(1):107-111

[6] Samson SL, Garber AJ. Metabolic syndrome (in eng). Endocrinology and Metabolism Clinics of North America. 2014;**43**(1):1-23

[7] Saklayen MG. The global epidemic of the metabolic syndrome. Current Hypertension Reports. 2018;**20**(2):12

[8] McCracken E, Monaghan M, Sreenivasan S. Pathophysiology of the metabolic syndrome (in eng). Clinics in Dermatology. 2018;**36**(1):14-20

[9] Roberts CK, Hevener AL, Barnard RJ. Metabolic syndrome and insulin resistance: Underlying causes and modification by exercise training (in eng). Comprehensive Physiology. 2013;**3**(1):1-58

[10] Kishida K, Funahashi T, Matsuzawa Y, Shimomura I. Visceral adiposity as a target for the management of the metabolic syndrome (in eng). Annals of Medicine. 2012;**44**(3): 233-241

[11] Raal FJ. Pathogenesis and management of the dyslipidemia of the metabolic syndrome, (in eng). Metabolic Syndrome and Related Disorders. 2009;**7**(2):83-88

[12] Capasso R, Izzo AA, Pinto L, Bifulco T, Vitobello C, Mascolo N. Phytotherapy and quality of herbal medicines (in eng). Fitoterapia. 2000;**71**(Suppl. 1):S58-S65

[13] Kumar S, Mittal A, Babu D, Mittal A. Herbal medicines for diabetes management and its secondary complications (in eng). Current Diabetes Reviews. 2021;**17**(4):437-456

[14] Eckel RH, Grundy SM, Zimmet PZ. The metabolic syndrome (in eng). Lancet. 2005;**365**(9468):1415-1428

[15] Payab M et al. Effect of the herbal medicines in obesity and metabolic syndrome: A systematic review and meta-analysis of clinical trials (in eng). Phytotherapy Research. 2020;**34**(3):526-545

[16] Nouri Z, Hajialyani M, Izadi Z, Bahramsoltani R, Farzaei MH, Abdollahi M. Nanophytomedicines for the prevention of metabolic syndrome: A pharmacological and biopharmaceutical review (in eng). Frontiers in Bioengineering and Biotechnology. 2020;**8**:425-425

[17] Sanati S, Razavi BM, Hosseinzadeh H. A review of the

effects of *Capsicum annuum* L. and its constituent, capsaicin, in metabolic syndrome (in eng). Iranian Journal of Basic Medical Sciences. 2018;**21**(5):439-448

[18] Razavi BM, Hosseinzadeh H. Saffron: A promising natural medicine in the treatment of metabolic syndrome (in eng). Journal of the Science of Food and Agriculture. 2017;**97**(6):1679-1685

[19] Shakib Z, Shahraki N, Razavi BM, Hosseinzadeh H. Aloe vera as an herbal medicine in the treatment of metabolic syndrome: A review (in eng). Phytotherapy Research. 2019;**33**(10):2649-2660

[20] Xie W, Zhao Y, Zhang Y. Traditional chinese medicines in treatment of patients with type 2 diabetes mellitus (in eng). Evidence-based Complementary and Alternative Medicine. 2011;**2011**:726723

[21] Wang J, Xiong X. Outcome measures of chinese herbal medicine for hypertension: An overview of systematic reviews. Evidence-based Complementary and Alternative Medicine. 2012;**2012**:697237

[22] Aminifard T, Razavi BM, Hosseinzadeh H. The effects of ginseng on the metabolic syndrome: An updated review (in eng). Food Science & Nutrition. 2021;**9**(9):5293-5311

[23] Nyakudya TT, Tshabalala T, Dangarembizi R, Erlwanger KH, Ndhlala AR. The potential therapeutic value of medicinal plants in the management of metabolic disorders. Molecules. 2020;**25**(11):2669

[24] Aziz TA, Hussain SA, Mahwi TO, Ahmed ZA, Rahman HS, Rasedee A. The efficacy and safety of Ginkgo biloba extract as an adjuvant in type 2 diabetes mellitus patients ineffectively managed with metformin: A double-blind, randomized, placebo-controlled trial (in eng). Drug Design, Development and Therapy. 2018;**12**:735-742

Chapter 7

Intervention for the Prevention of Lifestyle-Related Diseases in Healthy Japanese Residents

Masayo Nagai

Abstract

Lifestyle-related diseases can reduce their risk by improving their lives. Therefore, various efforts are being made, such as health education, to prevent lifestyle-related diseases. However, lifestyles are complicated and their prevention is not easy. Local residents who are active in health promotion are often working to improve their lifestyles. It is possible for residents to have excessive expectations for disease prevention simply by changing their lifestyles, paying attention only to the limited aspects of their lifestyles. However, if you pay attention to only one point and lack consideration for the whole, you cannot always expect the effect of lifestyle-related improvement. Therefore, it is necessary to understand how the subject perceives his/her lifestyle. This is also important for continued intervention. In addition, it is necessary to examine how health consciousness is related to the parameters of lifestyle-related diseases in such a health-conscious group. In this chapter, we would like to discuss the previously reported reports on the awareness of local residents regarding the prevention of lifestyle-related diseases, the need for health counseling, and issues in future efforts.

Keywords: lifestyle, lifestyle-related diseases, prevention, awareness of prevention, local residents

1. Introduction

The risk of lifestyle-related diseases can be reduced if a favorable lifestyle is followed, and various activities, such as education to promote health, have been performed to prevent such diseases [1–4]. Regional needs for health consultation have elevated with increases in the incidences of lifestyle-related diseases [5]. In community infirmaries located at places different from medical institutions, counseling involving prevention or information on medical practice, nursing, and health are provided, considering the region and family [6]. Regional health consultation may play many roles, such as health maintenance/promotion, disease prevention, and the early detection of abnormalities.

However, lifestyle is associated with a variety of individuals' daily lives, and it is not easy to prevent lifestyle-related diseases. A study investigated the association of lifestyle, including diet, with the degree of arteriosclerosis, visceral fat level, and bone mineral density (BMD) as an attempt to prevent lifestyle-related diseases in regional residents, and indicated that, in addition to the frequency of consuming various foods, the meal style was more strongly associated with lifestyle-related diseases [1], suggesting the necessity of guidance regarding personal lifestyle-matched diet. A survey regarding the relationship between exercise and parameters of lifestyle-related diseases [7] involved residents with positive attitudes toward health promotion, but exercise was not always positively correlated with parameters of lifestyle-related diseases. These studies suggest that complex factors are involved in lifestyle-related diseases, and that exercise alone does not absolutely reduce such diseases.

Many regional residents with positive attitudes toward health promotion make efforts to review their lifestyle [5]. Residents who are aware of lifestyle-related disease prevention may excessively expect disease prevention by lifestyle modification from a limited aspect alone. However, if consideration for the whole is absent, the effects of lifestyle improvement may not always be obtained. The risk of lifestyle-related diseases successively increases, and we cannot conclude that values above the reference range reflect the risk, whereas values below it reflect the safety. Therefore, it is important for residents after measurement to review their health or lifestyle regardless of the results of the measurement [2]. It is advantageous to understand how they recognize their own lifestyle for continuous intervention. Furthermore, few studies have examined how health consciousness is associated with parameters of lifestyle-related diseases in such a population with high-level health consciousness.

In this chapter, we introduce a previous report on regional residents' recognition regarding the prevention of lifestyle-related diseases [2] and analysis of previous results, and examine the needs for health consultation and issues for future attempts.

2. Lifestyle consciousness

According to a survey regarding Japanese people's awareness of health, 73.7% of the subjects selected "very healthy" or "slightly healthy" with respect to their health status [8]. Furthermore, persons undergoing a health checkup in the general areas of Japan are health-conscious, and many persons are positively doing health behaviors [9]. A study indicated that the levels of health consciousness and attitudes in persons who have not undergone a health checkup were lower than in those undergoing it and that the rate of persons who do not perform health habits was higher [10]. However, knowledge about a healthy lifestyle alone does not lead to an improvement in lifestyle [11]. If recognition regarding lifestyle is confirmed on measurement of parameters of lifestyle-related diseases, this may lead to an improvement in awareness of lifestyle, including diet and physical activities [1]. A previous study [2] examined how regional residents understand their health or lifestyle and whether these factors are associated with the speed of sound (SOS), arterial stiffness (acceleration plethysmography: APG), and visceral fat area (VFA) as parameters of lifestyle-related diseases.

With respect to the results of SOS, APG, and VFA measurement, multiple regression analysis with a questionnaire regarding lifestyle showed that there was no factor associated with these parameters. However, this previous study indicated that some recognitions regarding health or lifestyle were associated with age. In particular, in persons of more advanced age, the rate of those who are satisfied with their health management was higher (**Table 1**). It is known that there are differences in health behaviors among ages. According to a report from the Ministry of Health, Labour and Welfare [8], in persons aged ≥65 years, the number of matters for which they work

	Age			
	Men and Women		Women	
	β	P-value	β	P-value
Do you think that your health management is appropriate?	0.257	0.002*	0.180	0.039*
Do you have someone to alleviate your worries to promote your health and its management?	−0.195	0.016*	−0.315	<0.000*
Do you think that natural physical constitution greatly affects disorder?	−0.153	0.133	−0.112	0.325
Do you think that the physical constitution is an inheritance from a parent?	−0.002	0.982	−0.029	0.799
Do you think that exercise and nutrients only play a secondary role in health?	0.117	0.161	0.238	0.006*
Do you think that arteriosclerosis is a disorder?	0.056	0.496	0.071	0.401
Do you think that osteoporosis is a disorder?	−0.048	0.616	<0.000	0.998
Do you think that obesity is a disorder?	−0.247	0.012*	−0.298	0.004*
Do you think that arteriosclerosis is by nature?	0.035	0.722	0.101	0.337
Do you think that osteoporosis is by nature?	0.014	0.88	0.034	0.721
Do you think that obesity is by nature?	−0.124	0.786	−0.194	0.045*
Multiple correlation coefficient	0.494		0.579	
Coefficient of determination	0.244		0.335	
F-value significance	<0.000		<0.001	

P-value less than 0.05 were considered statistically significant and shown in the symbol followed (*). The statistical significance of the questionnaire responses was evaluated by multiple regression analysis. Dependent variable was age. Independent variables were index regarding the subjects' awareness of health and lifestyle.
Reproduced from reference Nagai [2].

Table 1.
Independent factors contributing to age.

actively or to which they pay attention for health promotion and lifestyle-related factors which they are aware of was larger than in other younger age groups. Furthermore, another survey involving Japanese with respect to age showed that the rate of persons practicing all items of lifestyle, and being aware of a healthy lifestyle, in those aged ≥45 years was higher than in those aged <45 years [12]. Another study indicated that the rate of awareness of the importance of physical activities and diet was high in ≥65-year-old persons participating in an exercise class, whereas that for physical-activity- and diet-based health promotion was low in such persons aged 45 to 64 years [13]. The rate of persons who are mindful of their health increases with age [5].

Each person's or his/her family's/friend's experience with illness related to aging increases anxiety about health. This may contribute to interests in health emerging with age. Furthermore, many participants in our previous study [2] had retired from work. Having time to spare may also be a factor for interests in health [14].

In our population in which the level of health consciousness may be high, consisting of those independently participating in a regional health checkup, it was also confirmed that there was a close association between age and degree of satisfaction with health management [2]. Furthermore, the subjects of this previous study [2]

	28 men		152 women	
	Average	±SD	Average	±SD
Age (y)	64.78	8.72	55.47	14.01
BMI (kg/m^2)	23.75	2.40	22.34	3.27
APG (m/s)	0.06	0.26	0.08	0.31
SOS (m/s)*	1517.10	30.74	1518.62	42.12
VFA (cm^2)**	96.32	26.92	70.86	24.97

BMD (Bone Mineral Density) estimated by SOS.
**VFA (visceral fat area) measured by BIA (bioelectrical impedance).*
BMI: body mass index, APG: arterial stiffness measured using acceleration plethysmography, SOS: sound of speed, VFA: visceral fat area.
Reproduced from reference Nagai [2].

Table 2.
Mean and range of each parameter in healthy subjects.

were 180 healthy adults (28 males and 152 females); the rate of females was higher (**Table 2**). When analyzing the females alone, the degree of satisfaction with health management also significantly increased with age. Previous studies indicated that the level of health consciousness in females was higher than in males [15, 16]. In particular, Japanese females more frequently play roles, such as domestic affairs, childcare, and nursing, at home compared with males. Therefore, there may be more opportunities to think about lifestyle or health.

On the other hand, it was shown that it was more difficult to obtain social support at a more advanced age [2]. The results suggest that the number of surrounding people who can hear about anxiety has decreased despite aging-related increases in health consciousness and interest in diseases; the role of a health checkup as a social resource may be important. Many males answered that they consulted the attending physician about diseases, whereas ≥40% of females did not have any attending physician. This may be because, in females, the rate of those belonging to companies is lower than in males. A previous study [9] also indicated that ≥50% of females who have not undergone a health checkup were unemployed. Furthermore, it was reported that the quality of life (QOL) was better for those receiving more human support [17], and a strong relationship among residents improved the health checkup rate [9]. Social capitals are associated with lifestyle or health behaviors.

Concerning the understanding of lifestyle-related diseases, most persons recognized arteriosclerosis and osteoporosis as diseases, whereas the rate of those recognizing obesity as a disease decreased with age (**Table 1**). It was shown that the rate of persons who do not recognize obesity as a disease despite awareness of health or diseases was high in elderly persons [2]. Healthy participants may not feel disease morbidity, seriousness, or threat at the present stage [5]. People can imagine the association of arteriosclerosis with cerebrovascular or heart diseases and that of osteoporosis with serious circumstances, such as a bedridden state related to fracture-prone features. However, obesity is more strongly associated with males, and this may have influenced the above finding.

The previous study [2] indicated that age was associated with some health consciousness items and health behaviors. In a health-conscious population, it was necessary to provide necessary information or motivation for continuation, suggesting the necessity of future continuous intervention. In addition, how these recognitions change through the provision of information or individual health consultation on participation in a health checkup and which type of information provision or health consultation is necessary must be examined.

3. Parameters of lifestyle-related diseases in the persons who continuously participate in a health check

For the prevention of lifestyle-related diseases, it is important to continue a healthy lifestyle. However, it was reported that lifestyle-related diseases gradually progressed in a long lifestyle history with no symptoms, not leading to behavioral changes [18, 19]. The effects of changing lifestyles, such as exercise and diet, may be obtained if it is continued for a long period. However, discontinuation results in ineffectiveness, and long-term continuation is difficult [20–22]. In addition, control is difficult, [23], raising issues. Furthermore, few studies have reported continuous support [24]. On the other hand, continuous intervention reduces the risk of lifestyle-related diseases. It was reported that long-term intervention influenced cardiovascular health parameters [25].

A previous cross-sectional study clarified that the mode of diet was more strongly associated with parameters of lifestyle-related diseases in regional residents positively participating in a health checkup [1]. In this chapter, we investigated the effects of continuous participation on changes in parameters of lifestyle-related diseases in healthy regional residents, continuously participating in a health checkup, who did not report the results again among the subjects of the previous study [1].

Two hundred and eighty-nine residents participated in health consultation in our previous study [1]. Of these, 30 (10.4%, 4 males, and 26 females) were continuous participants. During the 1.5-year study period, the mean frequency of participation in health consultation was 3.6 times, and the mean interval of participation was 3.5 months. The contents of participation consisted of measurement of the arterial stiffness, BMD, and VFA, as parameters of lifestyle-related diseases, and a questionnaire survey regarding lifestyle. The study subjects explained the results of measurement, and health consultation regarding lifestyle was possible [1].

In this chapter, we reviewed changes in the participants' lifestyles or parameters of lifestyle-related diseases. We analyzed the changes between the first and second sessions of participation and between the second and third sessions of participation. As a result, there was a significant decrease in the body mass index (BMI) between the first and second sessions of participation in health consultation ($p = 0.068$). There were no changes in the other parameters (BMD, VFA, and arterial stiffness). Based on the responses to a questionnaire, there was no change in lifestyle.

Participation in health consultation was optional, and the subjects of this study may be health-conscious, and living a healthy life. In the study subjects, a decrease in BMI after participation in health consultation was confirmed; health consultation may be an opportunity for further motivation. BMI decreases with weight loss, and this may have contributed to the confirmation of its decrease during a period of 1.5 years. However, arteriosclerosis progresses with age even in healthy adults [26]; therefore, it may have been difficult to examine changes during the previous study period.

In future, a long-term continuous survey may clarify changes in parameters of lifestyle-related diseases, which may not change in a short period, and daily lifestyle. Furthermore, it was reported that the health checkup and screening rates were low in persons who participated in health consultation for the first time and those who participated to measure health indices [27]. It is necessary to comprehensively support personal health or life in addition to measurement.

4. Needs for measurement of parameters of lifestyle-related diseases

Previously, we reported that health-conscious persons positively participated in health checkups [1, 2]. Furthermore, strongly motivated persons may achieve an improvement in lifestyle more readily [28]. It is important to recognize the results of measurement by participating in a health checkup, and this may lead to interest in health management, motivating individuals to improve their lifestyle. In the participants in health checkups in the previous studies [1, 2], a questionnaire survey regarding needs for measurement was conducted, but the results are not presented. In this chapter, we report the data through further validation.

Most subjects who participated in the previous studies positively accepted the measurement of parameters of lifestyle-related diseases (**Figure 1**). In addition, there was a description that measurement or its results might be utilized for future health management or lifestyle improvement. Of the subjects, ≥90% wished to measure these parameters in the future. As the most frequent reason, they wished for health management (**Table 3**). A study regarding health-checkup-undergoing behaviors [9] also indicated that the primary purpose of undergoing a health checkup was "health management."

Furthermore, our data showed that there was no significant association between the motivation for measurement and parameters of lifestyle-related diseases. It was also confirmed that the rate of persons wishing measurement differed among relevant diseases. Concerning measurement of the degree of arteriosclerosis, many persons wished to measure it; they may imagine the risk of cerebrovascular/cardiovascular diseases. Furthermore, the number of those wishing for BMD measurement was large. This was possible because many female participants considered the risk of fracture.

The visualization of lifestyle parameters through these measurements allows participating residents to maintain the goal of preventive attempts or motivation. Furthermore, several residents answered that they wished for measurement due to anxiety; measurement may play a role in relieving anxiety about health. A previous study [29] also reported that the rate of persons who are anxious about the results of measurement was higher in those recognizing a lower BMD and that the rate of those making efforts to increase the BMD was higher. It was indicated that recognition of the results of BMD measurement led to the opportunity of being interested in health management or efforts to improve lifestyle, resulting in the prevention of osteoporosis. Lifestyle, including diet and physical activities, may be improved through BMD measurement [30]. Furthermore, it was reported that habitual tooth brushing contributed to attention to health or consciousness, inhibiting an increase in the BMI or abdominal circumference [31]. Participation in a health checkup and measurement of physical data may be useful for providing motivation for primary prevention under interests in health or improving the QOL.

In addition, a study indicated that, after subjects received health guidance regarding the prevention of lifestyle-related diseases, approximately 30% of their family members felt favorable changes regarding health [32]. Furthermore, there was a significant difference in the age in the group with family changes, and elderly persons may have had time to spare. Among the subjects who participated in our survey, the rate of elderly subjects was high, and similar effects may be obtained.

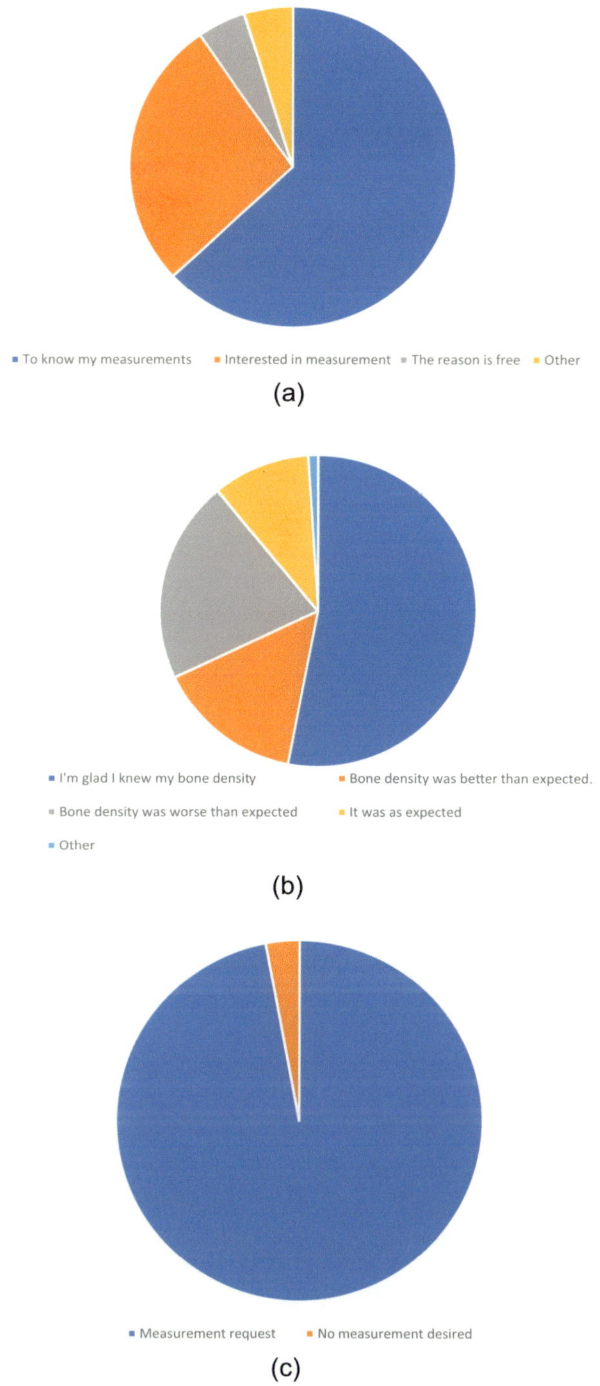

Figure 1.
A. Reason for measuring calcaneal ultrasonic propagation velocity. The reason for participating in the calcaneal ultrasonic propagation velocity measurement was shown (N = 206). B. Reaction by receiving bone density measurement. Impressions after participating in bone density measurement were shown (N = 205). C. Needs for bone density measurement. Results of asking for participation in regular bone mineral density measurements are shown (N = 205).

Reasons for requesting bone Density measurement	N*	Reasons for requesting arteriosclerosis measurement	N*
Health management	41	Health management	33
Confirm the effect of lifestyle-related correction	24	Confirm the effect of lifestyle-related correction	8
Anxiety	18	Anxiety	12
Disease prevention /early detection	7	Disease prevention /early detection	6
Other: If there is an opportunity	9	Other: If there is an opportunity	4
Reasons for not requesting to measure bone density	N	Reasons for not requesting to measure arteriosclerosis	N
Measured at the hospital on a regular basis	1	Unconcerned	2
Unconcerned	3	I do not want to change my eating habits	1
No time	1	No time	1
No opportunity	1		

**N means the number of respondents.*

Table 3.
Reasons for requesting to measure.

In this chapter, we again confirmed regional residents' needs for the measurement of lifestyle-related disease-associated parameters in health consultation. An opportunity to review lifestyle, including diet and physical activities, may be provided through these measurements, leading to lifestyle improvement. Such measurements are useful as a motivation for health promotion. Regular measurements may contribute to the maintenance of subjects' and their families' motivations to make efforts for health promotion.

5. Needs of behavioral changes to prevent lifestyle-related diseases

To promote behavioral changes, a clear motivation, high feasibility, and the absence of resistance are necessary. Stress in daily living hinders behavioral practice [24]. Thus, mental factors may be closely related to the improvement of lifestyle-related behaviors. Among these factors, it is useful to improve confidence in self-management behaviors and self-efficacy as a recognition of self-potential [33]. When lifestyle correction is difficult in high-risk patients for atherosclerotic cardiovascular diseases (ASCVDs), such as dyslipidemia and hypertension, the difficulty is related to a reduction in self-efficacy or its disappearance in many cases [34]. To improve self-efficacy, support by health care professionals and subjective life management are important [24, 33]. However, there is no fact that the values of lifestyle parameters are better in persons who are more strongly aware of a healthy lifestyle [2]. When improvement effects are not obtained, there may be a reduction in self-efficacy for the following reasons: the lifestyle improvement-related amelioration of test results leads to a sense of accomplishment, improving self-efficacy [35]; and test result-based confirmation alone is possible during the symptom-free period [19].

On the other hand, many regional residents who positively attempt to promote health have positively reviewed exercise and diet [15]. It is speculated that participants in health checkups or classes may essentially maintain a healthy lifestyle [1, 5, 10, 36]. According to a study, there was no change in the parameter of arteriosclerosis despite a change in lifestyle in some patients in whom the parameter was within the normal range before intervention [37]. Furthermore, a study [38] examined the influence of health education regarding the prevention of arteriosclerosis on health behaviors and indicated that there might have been no behavioral change due to the essentially high health behavior level of the subjects. In subjects who positively attempt to promote health, there may be no lifestyle-change-related improvement in the test results. Concerning the BMD and degree of vascular aging, even the maintenance of the status quo is sometimes evaluated as effective, considering aging [1].

Furthermore, the number of male participants was small during these health checkups. Another previous study also indicated that the number of male participants was small. Support for subjects who do not participate in the field of health promotion is emphasized as an issue [5]. In males, the presence of a spouse is a factor that promotes participation in a health checkup. In those without a spouse living together, encouragement by their families, close friends, or neighbors, who replace a spouse, is effective [9]. Among the participants in health checkups, there were many males participating at their spouses' invitation. Approaches to share health promotion with family members are also necessary.

According to the Comprehensive Survey of Living Conditions [39], the most frequent reasons why a health checkup or screening was skipped were "no time" and "expenditure." In the participant questionnaire we conducted, "free" was one of the reasons for wanting to receive the measurement. Participants answered that they did not want to measure in the future because they did not have time (**Table 3** and **Figure 2**). Furthermore, the absence of symptoms leads to a low lifestyle-related disease-associated health checkup rate in some cases [9, 40]. On regional health checkups, the free measurement may be available in a short time; this may be useful for maintaining health management behaviors. Concerning the absence of symptoms, visualization with parameters of lifestyle-related diseases may contribute to health management.

Persons utilizing regional health consultation answered that "counter consultation by medical specialists" was necessary to resolve anxiety or doubts about health [5]. A survey involving subjects who have not utilized regional health consultation [41] showed that even non-users highly recognized the necessity of health consultation. The contents of the needs included feeling free to consult a nurse as a specialist in the home city, free consultation, and attempts for individuality-emphasized continuous support. For lifestyle management, it is important to recognize individual problems and hear about various living conditions as the role of nursing [42].

The subjects who cooperated in our study had independently participated in health consultation; they may have comprised a health-conscious population. The participants may also require support from medical specialists. It is necessary to continue support for subjective attempts under specialists' assistance. Furthermore, the effects of group guidance may not appear if there is no merit in changing lifestyle. It is difficult to change lifestyle [43]. The presence of a place for individual consultation based on active participation may be important to change behaviors or maintain health behaviors.

However, lifestyle is an extremely private matter, and interference by other persons leads to uncomfortableness [44]. Excessive intervention may result in stress loading for healthy adults, inducing an unhealthy state through obesity, or an increase in the alcohol volume [45]. We can imagine that compulsive lifestyle intervention by other persons markedly reduces the mental QOL. For exercise support to improve the

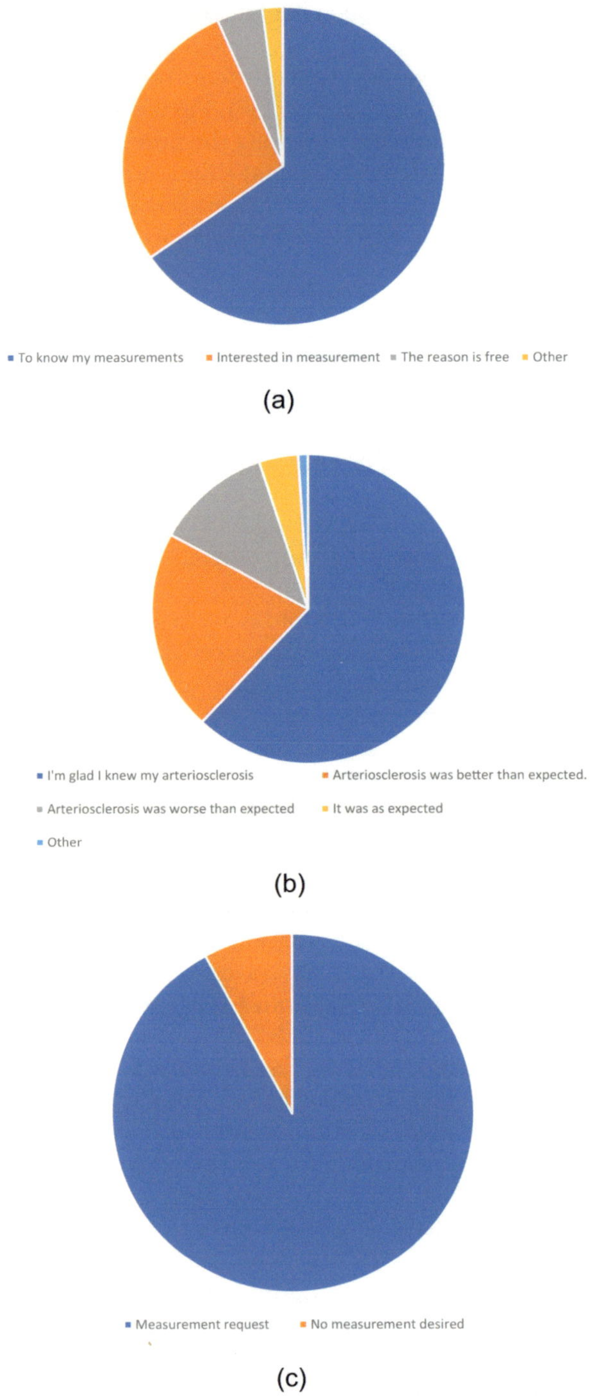

Figure 2.
A. Reason for measuringarteriosclerosis. The reason for participating in the arteriosclerosis measurement was shown (N = 150). B. Reaction by arteriosclerosis measurement. Impressions after participating in arteriosclerosis measurement were shown (N = 145). C. Needs for arteriosclerosis measurement. Results of asking for participation in regular arteriosclerosis measurements are shown (N = 144).

QOL, the intensity of exercise and subjectivity should be valued [37]. The purpose of health checkups is to improve participants' QOL through the prevention of lifestyle-related diseases. For support to improve lifestyle, it may also be important to value individuals' subjectivity based on scientific evidence.

6. Conclusions

Even subjects with a healthy life have needs for attempts to prevent lifestyle-related diseases under specialists' support. In particular, aging increases health consciousness or interest in diseases, but there are few familiar persons to consult in some cases. Also, obesity should be recognized as a disease. Regional health consultation and measurement of parameters of lifestyle-related diseases by nurses are important for living toward prevention and continuous support. Lifestyle-related parameter measurements also have the purpose of maintaining an ongoing motivation for health care. For participants, this is an opportunity to review their lifestyle, being useful for individuals' health promotion. In addition, an approach to enhance self-efficacy is important for improving lifestyle to prevent lifestyle-related diseases.

Acknowledgements

The study was supported by volunteer participants and nurses.

Also, the study was supported by Grant-in-Aid for Scientific Research from JSPS KAKENHI Grant Number JP20K23147 and JP22K17448.

Conflict of interest

The authors have declared that no competing interests exist.

Author details

Masayo Nagai
Department of Nursing, Faculty of Health Science, Aino University, Japan

*Address all correspondence to: m-nagai@ns-u.aino.ac.jp

References

[1] Nagai M, Uyama O, Kaji H. Dietary habits prone to lifestyle-related disease. Health Education Journal. 2013;**72**(2):172-179. DOI: 10.1177/0017896912437299

[2] Nagai M. Relationships among lifestyle awareness, age, and lifestyle-related diseases in healthy Japanese community residents. Asian Pacific Island Nursing Journal. 2020;**5**(2): 103-110. DOI: 10.31372/20200502.1092 PMID: 33043138; PMCID: PMC7544015

[3] White ND, Lenz TL, Smith K. Tool guide for lifestyle behavior change in a cardiovascular risk reduction program. Psychology Research and Behavior Management. 2013;**6**:55-63

[4] King EL, Grunseit AC, O'Hara BJ, et al. Evaluating the effectiveness of an Australian obesity mass-media campaign: How did the 'Measure-Up' campaign measure up in New South Wales? Health Education Research. 2013;**28**:1029-1039

[5] Sasaki A, Watanabe M, Kawauchi K. Survey on the health of local residents. -through activities at Kenko booth. Mejiro Journal of Health Care Sciences. 2019;**12**:67-78

[6] Suzuki T, Teraura H, Manabe T, Kotani K. Characterisrics of two kinds of communitu-based healthcare rooms: A literature revier. Jichi Medical University Journal. 2019;**42**:47-56

[7] Nagai M, Uyama O, Kaji H. Daily physical activity and body composition in healthy Japanese women. Structure and Function. 2015;**13**(2):61-68

[8] Ministry of Health, Labour and Welfare. Annual Report on Health, Labour and Welfare. 2014. 1-02-1.pdf (mhlw.go.jp)

[9] Imoto C, Yamada K, Morioka I. The association of Japan's specific medical checkup with a health promotion lifestyle, health literacy, and social capital by healthcare coverage type. Japanese Society of Public Health. 2019;**66**(6):295-305

[10] Fuchino Y. A study on the relationship between working peoples' health awareness and their life habits. Bulletin of the School of Nursing, Yamaguchi Prefectural University. 2002;**6**:63-67

[11] Nanri A, Matsushita Y, Ichikawa F, Yamamoto M, Kakumoto Y, Mizoue T. Effect of six months lifestyle intervention in Japanese men with metabolic syndrome randomized controlled trial. Journal of Occupational Health. 2012;**54**:215-222

[12] Kimura M, Endo H, Hiruma M. Bone mineral density, dietary habits, and exercise habit in adult women: Results of osteoporosis screaning in kyoto prefecture. Bulletin of College of Medical Technology Kyoto Prefectural University of Medicine. 1999;**8**:107-116

[13] Oyama K, Sakuyama M. Investigation of physical fitness and life style of middle-aged participants on a sporting activities course (I). Annual Report of Iwate Medical University School of Liberal Arts and Sciences. 2002;**37**:121-126

[14] Tsushita K et al. Evaluation of physical activity of diabetic patients by using the pedometer with large memory accelerometer. Journal of the Japan Diabetes Society. 1999;**42**(4):289-297

[15] Fukatsu C, Sakamoto K. A study on the dietary habits of aged and young people. Sonoda Journal. 1993;**28**:147-160

[16] Nagasawa N, Kondo U, Nakajima J. The relationship between obesity, health examination results, health-consciousness and life-style. Journal of Nagoya Women's University, Home Economics Natural Science. 1997;**43**:91-100

[17] Morimoto K, Maruyama S. Lifestyle and physical and mental health. Japanese Journal of Psychosomatic Medicine. 2001;**41**:241-251

[18] Goto M, Tanaka M. Issues related to health support for elderly people in an intermediate and mountainous area: Results from health consultation by nursing students. (Abstract in English). Archives of Yamaguchi Prefectural University. 2012;**5**:11-19

[19] Tsushita K, Muramoto A, Kato A. Lifestyle guidance for troubled patients. (the title is translated by the author) case 01-05. Japanese Medical Journal. 2014;**4722**:16-39

[20] Soyano A, Momose Y, Watanabe M, Izawa M, Yokoyama Y, Murakami M. Evaluation on exercise adherence of two health promotion programs. Journal of Physical Education and Medicine. 2005;**7**:7-14

[21] Shibuya K et al. The adherence and long-term effect after one year of bench step exercise program for prevention and/or improvement of lifestyle related disease. Ningen Dock. 2008;**23**(1):21-26

[22] Tsushita K. Prospective view for the next version of specific health check-up and health guidance system, based on the performance evaluation for eight years. Ningen Dock. 2016;**31**:7-21

[23] Kuno S, Tanabe K, Yoshizawa H. Significance of exercise for prevention of lifestyle-related diseases and importance of environmental measures to make it feasible. (the title is translated by the author). Journal of the Society of Biomechanisms. 2011;**35**(2):91-97

[24] Takagi E, Yamaguchi K, Tomita S, Kimura M. Qualitative study on factors in promoting Behavioral changes through continuous support in specific health guidance for metabolic syndrome. Ningen Dock. 2009;**24**(4):35-39

[25] Devaraj SM, Rockette-Wagner B, Miller RG, et al. The impact of a yearlong diabetes prevention program-based lifestyle intervention on cardiovascular health metrics. Journal of Primary Care and Community Health. 2021;**12**:21501327211029816. DOI: 10.1177/21501327211029816

[26] Redheuil A, Yu WC, Wu CO, Mousseaux E, de Cesare A, Yan R, et al. Reduced ascending aortic strain and distensibility: Earliest manifestations of vascular aging in humans. Hypertension. 2010;**55**(2):319-326. DOI: 10.1161/HYPERTENSIONAHA.109.141275

[27] Matsui N et al. Health status and health behavior of local residents attending "Machi no Hokenshitsu" at Mukogawa Women's University School of Nursing. Nursing Journal of Mukogawa Women's University. 2021;**6**:79-89

[28] Kadoma A, Shirai M. Achievement motive and its application to nursing. A review based on motivation for health-educatee and nurses. Journal of Nagoya Women's university, home economics. Natural Science. 2002;**2**:21-27

[29] Ikeda J, Higashi A, Watanabe Y, Matsumura A, Sugino S, Honjo H. The relation of consciousness of bone mineral density to the changes in daily dietary habits and daily behaviors. Japanese Society of Public Health. 1999;**46**(7):569-578

[30] Naka T, Nakajima D, Tae-Wong OH, Illyoung HAN, Sakurai T, Igawa S.

Effects of lifestyle on bone metabolism in middle-aged and aged Japanese wome. Journal of Physiological Anthropology. 2004;**9**(3):1-9

[31] Wada T et al. Living conditions of obese people -analysis by 22 living factors (the title is translated by the author). Journal of Japan Society for the Study of Obesity. 2004;**10**(3):282-286

[32] Kiryu I, Sato Y. Dose receiving health guidance concerning lifestyle-related disease prevention affect the health of the participant's family? Japanese Journal of Research in Family Nursing. 2019;**24**(2):156-163

[33] Sugunari Y, Izumino K, Sawada A, Takama S. Factor influencing management behavior and self-efficacy in outpatients with cardiovascular disease. The Journal of the Nursing Society of the Toyama Medical and Pharmaceutical University. 2002;**4**(2):21-31

[34] Kimura Y. Cognitive behavior therapy for the patients with diabetes and obesity. Japanese Journal of General Hospital Psychiatry. 2011;**23**(4):348-354

[35] Murakami M, Umeki S, Hanada T. The factors promoting and hindering the self-care of patients with diabetes. Japanese Journal of Nursing Research. 2009;**32**(4):29-38

[36] Tsushita K. The effects of lifestyle intervention on obesity diseases. The Journal of the Japan Medical Association. 2014;**143**(1):49-53

[37] Yamada E, Aoki H, Shimizu U, Muramatsu Y. Pilot study on the effects of 3 months of exercise and movement to increase physical flexibility, selected mainly by patients with middle-aged female hypertension, on arteriosclerosis-related indicators and health-related quality of life. Journal of Japanese Society for Chronic Illness and Conditions Nursing. 2019;**13**(2):91-98

[38] Hayashi S, Kawata C. Effect of behavioral modification through health education on arteriosclerosis prevention. The Journal of Nursing Investigation. 2010;**9**(1):20-26

[39] Ministry of Health, Labour and Welfare. National Health and Nutrition Survey. 2017. Available from: https://www.nibiohn.go.jp/eiken/english/research/project_nhns.html

[40] Ogawa M, Ito K, Kato T. Present situation and future issues of follow-up after health check-ups at our institute. Ningen Dock. 2019;**34**(3):443-449

[41] Fukui S, Otoguro C, Ishikawa T, Fujita J, Akiyama M. The need for health consultation services and related factors among non-users of health consultation services residing in urban public apartment complexes. Japanese Society of Public Health. 2013;**60**(12):745-753

[42] Banning M. The management of obesity: The role of the specialist nurse. British Journal of Nursing (Mark Allen Publishing). 2005;**14**:139-144

[43] Inoue R, Hihara Y, Inoue K, Nakagawa M. Efforts to motivate changes in perceptions and behaviors regarding exercise -started health guidance for accommodation dock examinees- (the title is translated by the author). NIHONKANGOGAKKAI RONNBUNSYU. 2012;**42**:132-134

[44] Kawata C. Aiming for evidence-based diabetes education efforts (the title is translated by the author). Journal of Japan Academy of Diabetes Education and Nursing. 2002;**6**(1):15-21

[45] Morimoto K. Environmental factor and Japanese people: Eight health practices as an index of lifestyle. 2022;**57**:680-688

Chapter 8

The Use of Waterpipe Tobacco Products and Its Associated Risk Factors among University of Limpopo Students, South Africa

Kotsedi Daniel Monyeki, Hlengani James Siweya and Phut Johanna Makgae

Abstract

The use of tobacco products is a modifiable risk factor for non-communicable diseases. The aim of the study was to determine the prevalence of waterpipe tobacco product use and associated risk factors amongst University of Limpopo students aged 17–43 years. This cross-sectional study comprises 916 (415 males and 501 females) University of Limpopo students aged 17–43 years. The questionnaire was validated for the University of Limpopo student population before it was used. Logistic regression was used to determine the associated risk factors for waterpipe tobacco product use among the University of Limpopo students. Staying on campus (OR 2.54 95%CI 1.87 3.44) or off-campus (0.39 95%CI 0.29 0.54) was significantly ($p<0.05$) associated with using waterpipe tobacco products even after adjusting for age and gender and receiving a bursary (on Campus OR=3.8095%CI 2.59 5.57) off-campus (0.26 95%CI 0.18 0.39). Our results demonstrate that waterpipe smoking was more prevalent among university male students than female students. Liking the taste and difficulties to refuse were significantly ($p<0.05$) associated with the use of waterpipe amongst University students. Future research should investigate the association of waterpipe use with risk factors for non-communicable diseases over time.

Keywords: waterpipe, NFSAS, current use, lifestyle, tobacco products university students

1. Introduction

Tobacco products have been widely reported all over the world in various populations with health effects as risk factors to non-communicable diseases [1]. By 2030, more than 80% of the deaths in developing countries could be accounted for by tobacco-related implications [2]. There are emerging methods of tobacco use that have become alarmingly common in specific population groups which include waterpipe tobacco use also referred to as hubbly bubbly, hooker, narguileh and shisha which comes in a variety of flavours such as mint, liquorice, strawberry, cappuccino and chocolate [3, 4]. Waterpipe (Hubbly bubbly, hooker, narguileh and shisha) is known by different titles depending on the segment of the globe it is being used as a form of tobacco delivery [4]. Briefly, 'the waterpipe instrument is set up with charcoal, filters, a bowl of water, rubber pipe and varying flavours'. The delivery of tobacco smoke moves through the rubber pipe attached to the bowl that directs large volumes of smoke inhaled into the mouth. Waterpipe smokers are exposed to the noxious materials of the tobacco smoke such as carbon monoxide, nitric oxide, nicotine, polycyclic aromatic hydrocarbons, nanoparticles, volatile aldehydes and furans [5]. Aboaziza and Eissenberg [6] reported that waterpipe smoking is associated with nicotine dependence and smoking-related diseases including cancer, cardiovascular disease, lung disease and adverse pregnancy outcomes. Students are knowledgeable about harmful health effects associated with waterpipe tobacco product use but continue to use it for a variety of reasons which include taste, peer pressure and easy availability [7]. Furthermore, university students regard waterpipe tobacco as a socially acceptable, popular, pleasant social experience and looks cooler than smoking cigarettes [8–10].

The prevalence of waterpipe smoking varies with areas of the world in student communities due to multifactorial influences [4]. A student study at the University of Beirut, Lebanon, reported 43% ever user and 28% of current smoking [2], while another study in the same country contrastingly reported current waterpipe use at 21% [11]. Kilic and Kasap [12] found in the American region 10% ever user and a 41% current use of waterpipe tobacco product use. In North Africa, it was found that men were four times most likely to report waterpipe smoking, with 64% of the sample investigated reporting long-term consumption [7]. In South Africa, waterpipe tobacco product use was reported to be 40% amongst Western Cape university students [7]. Van der Merwe *et al*, [13] reported 11% waterpipe tobacco product use among University of Cape Town students with social settings as the main reasons for using it. Furthermore, Miri-Moghaddam et al., [14] reported that friends played crucial roles in the high prevalence (78%) of waterpipe smoking amongst medical students in Iran.

University environments across the globe provide a unique opportunity for students to experiment with waterpipe tobacco smoking which can eventually become a lifelong use. However, little is known about the prevalence of waterpipe tobacco use amongst University of Limpopo students in the Limpopo province of South Africa. The study aimed to determine the prevalence of waterpipe tobacco products use and to investigate the associated risk factors amongst among University of Limpopo students aged 17–43 years.

2. Materials and methods

2.1 Geographical area

This cross-sectional study was carried out at the University of Limpopo, South Africa. The University of Limpopo is situated in the foothills of the Hwiti (Wolkberg range) in Mankweng Township (23.8837° S, 29.7079° E), midway between Polokwane and Magoebaskloof. It is a predominantly African ethnicity dominated student community. Most students come from low- and middle-income families and are receiving funding in the form of a government bursary called South African National Student Financial Aid Scheme (NSFAS). The students rely mostly on this NSFAS bursary scheme to cover their university expenses and other essentials.

2.2 Sampling procedure

Using STATA, the sample size required for the study was calculated based on a power of 80% and a two-tailed significance level of 5%, the prevalence of waterpipe smoking was 0.24% amongst university students with an alternative proportion of 20% [3, 15, 16].

A convenient sample of 916 students (415 males' mean age is 22.02 years, sd 2.97, and 501 females' mean age is 21.16, sd 2.71) aged 17–43 years, who were enrolled in all the faculties (Humanities, Health Sciences, Management and Law and Science and Agriculture) of the University of Limpopo in 2019 participated in this study.

2.3 Data collection

The questionnaire used in the present study was based on questions which have been used in the Ellisras Longitudinal Study and other studies [3, 15–17]. The questionnaire was shared with experts to ensure content, face and construct validity. It was then revised and piloted with a sample of students to make sure it was valid, reliable, acceptable and accurately understood.

The questionnaire comprised three sections. The first part of the questionnaire included information on age, sex, acquisition of NSFAS bursary, place of residence, the field of study, year of entering the university and the level of study. Briefly, current waterpipe smoker was defined as anyone who uses waterpipe tobacco products regularly or every day during the time of the survey. The following question was asked: 'Do you NOW use waterpipe regularly, at least once every day?' Ever waterpipe users were those who answered that they tried to use waterpipe tobacco products before the survey and have stopped, or they use them occasionally. The question used was: 'Have you ever used waterpipe to smoke (at least once)?' Those who had never used waterpipe tobacco products at the time of the survey were considered non-smokers., 'The onset (initiation age) age for waterpipe use was determined by the question "If yes, indicate how old you were when you first tried this____", How old were you when you first started using waterpipe tobacco everyday/regularly ______.'Onset age was the group as less than 20 years, between 21 and 25 years and over 26 years.

2.3.1 Educational achievements

Participants were asked to indicate their academic status ('first-year undergraduate' through to the third year, fourth year, master's and PhD). First and second-year undergraduates were combined to form 'lower level undergraduate' and third-year study was moderate to high level while fourth year, master's and PhD were grouped as a postgraduate level.

2.3.2 Social factors

Social factors for waterpipe tobacco products use were assessed with the following question: 'One smokes waterpipe tobacco products because I went with others having a good time and felt like inhaling and exhaling together (yes/no), One smokes waterpipe tobacco products because it is difficult to refuse (yes/no), waterpipe tobacco smoking helps me face a difficult situation with confidence (yes/no), One smokes waterpipe tobacco products because it gives me energy (yes/no), One smokes waterpipe tobacco products because I like the taste (yes/no)'.

The study received an ethical clearance from the University of Limpopo Ethics committee (TREC/61/2019: IR) before the data collection process commenced.

2.4 Statistical analysis

Descriptive statistics including frequency distributions and percentage frequencies were used to determine the prevalence of waterpipe tobacco product use among University of Limpopo students. A Chi-squared test was used to compare sets of nominal data that had larger frequency counts while the Fisher's exact test was used when frequency cells were small (less than five or ten) between genders [18, 19]. Logistic regression was used to determine the associated risk factors for waterpipe tobacco product use among the University of Limpopo students. All statistical analyses were performed using SPSS version 25. The statistical significance was set at $P< 0.05$.

3. Results

Figure 1 shows the prevalence of ever and current waterpipe use amongst University of Limpopo students. The prevalence of current waterpipe use was significantly ($p<0.05$) high (6.7%) for boys as compared with girls (3%) amongst the University of Limpopo students.

Table 1 shows the onset age and number of quitting attempts for water pipe use amongst University of Limpopo students aged 17–43 years. The prevalence of waterpipe tobacco product use for ever use in the onset age ranges between 1.6 and 3.9% for the age less than 20 years and between 17.8 and 26.7% for ages between 21 and 25 years. For the current waterpipe user, the prevalence was significantly ($p<0.05$) high 4.6% for boys as compared with 1.8% for girls between the ages of 21 and 25 years. It was clear from **Table 1** that 1.2% of the current boys who quit the use of waterpipe smoking lasted for more than a year. 4.6% of boys and 2.0% of girls never tried to quit using waterpipe smoking.

Table 2 presents the frequencies and percentage frequencies for a positive response for associated risk factors in using waterpipe tobacco amongst University of Limpopo students aged 17 to 43. A total of 70.6% of boys and 77% of girls stay on campus for the duration of their study while 29.4% of boys and 23% of girls stay

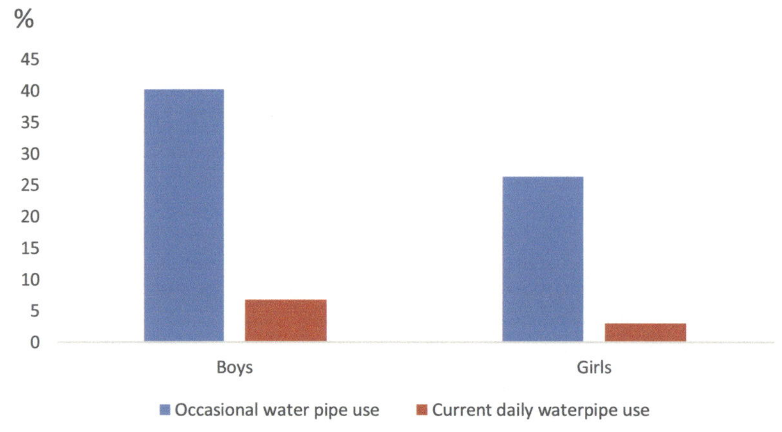

Figure 1.
Prevalence of occasional and current waterpipe use amongst University of Limpopo students.

	Boys N=415		Girls N=501	
	%	**(n)**	**%**	**(n)**
Ever water pipe use				
Less than 20 years	3.9	(16)	1.6	(8)
21 to 25 years	26.7*	(111)	17.6*	(88)
Over 26 years	9.6	(40)	7.2	(36)
Current water pipe use				
Less than 20 years	0.2	(1)	—	—
21 to 25 years	4.6*	(19)	1.8*	(9)
Over 26 years	1.9	(8)	1.2	(6)
Never tried to quit	4.6	(19)	2.0	(10)
Less than seven times a week	1.7	(7)	0.8	(4)
More than seven times a week	0.5	(2)	0.2	(1)
Less than a month	0.7	(3)	—	—
More than six months	0.5	(2)	0.8	(4)
More than a year	1.2	(5)	0.2	(1)

*=$p<0.05$.

Table 1.
Onset age and number of quitting attempts for waterpipe use amongst University of Limpopo students aged 17–43 years.

	Boys N=415		Girls N=501	
	%	**(n)**	**%**	**(n)**
Student residences				
On campus	70.6	(293)	77	(386)
Off-campus	29.4	(122)	23	(115)
Educational level				
Lower level	58.6	(235)	53.9	(270)
Moderate high level	23.1	(96)	25.5	(128)
Postgraduate level	20.2	(84)	20.6	(103)
Social factors				
Some smoke because they went with others having a good time and felt like inhaling and exhaling together	3.1*	(13)	0.2*	(1)
Some smoke because it is difficult to refuse	5.8*	(24)	1.6*	(8)
Some smoke because they like the taste	7.0	(29)	1.8	(9)
Some smoke because it gives them energy	10.6*	(44)	2.4*	(12)
Helps me face difficulties with confidence	6.0	(25)	2.4	(12)
Received NSFAS	71.8	(298)	80.2	(402)
Other bursaries than NSFAS	12.0	(50)	9.8	(49)

*=$p<0.05$.

Table 2.
Frequencies and percentage frequencies for a positive response for associated risk factors in using waterpipe tobacco amongst University of Limpopo students aged 17–43.

off-campus. A total of 5.8% boys and 1.6% girls who are currently using waterpipe smoking reported that it was difficult to refuse using waterpipe smoking while 7.0% of boys and 1.8% of girls reported that they like the taste of using waterpipe tobacco products, and the difference was significant (P<0.05).

Table 3 shows the logistic regression (odds ratio, 95%CI and P-value)) for the association between waterpipe tobacco product use and associated risk factors amongst University of Limpopo students aged 17–43 years. Older onset age (between 21 and 25 years (OR= 6.7 95%CI 3.63 13.05) and above 26 years (OR= 5.57 95%CI 2.77 11.21) was significantly associated with using waterpipe tobacco products even after adjusting for age, gender and receiving a bursary (21–25 years (OR- 6.98 95%CI 3.60, 13.54 and above 26 years (OR= 5.92 95%CI 2.81 12.49). Staying on campus (OR 2.54 95%CI 1.87 3.44) or off-campus (0.39 95%CI 0.29 0.54) was significantly (p<0.05)

	Unadjusted			**Adjusted for age, gender and receiving bursary***		
	OR	**P-value**	**(95%CI)**	**OR**	**P-value**	**95%CI**
Onset age						
Less than 20 years	0.88	0.902	(0.12 6.67)	0.70	0.731	(0.09 5.40)
20 to 25 years	6.87	0.000	(3.63 13.05)	6.98	0.000	(3.60 13.54)
Over 26 years	5.57	0.000	(2.77 11.21)	5.92	0.000	(2.81 12.49)
Number of times one tried to quit						
Never tried	7.81	0.000	(3.21 9.33)	9.04	0.000	(6.93 12.56)
Less than seven times	0.64	0.221	(0.31 0.86)	0.56	0.231	(0.21 0.96)
More than seven times	0.33	0.143	(0.21 1.37)	0.36	0.153	(0.11 0.95)
Student residence						
Off-Campus	2.54	0.000	(1.87 3.44)	3.80	0.000	(2.59 5.57)
On Campus	0.39	0.000	(0.29 0.54)	0.26	0.000	(0.18 0.39)
Educational level						
Lower level	0.84	0.211	(0.64 1.11)	0.74	0.051	(0.54 1.00)
Moderate high level	1.26	0.146	(0.92 1.73)	1.34	0.079	(0.97 1.85)
Postgraduate level	1.00	0.994	(0.71 1.41)	1.08	0.701	(0.74 1.56)
Social factors						
Went with others having a good time and felt like inhaling and exhaling together	7.98	0.066	(3.41 18.67)	7.19	0.072	(3.04 16.99)
One smokes because it is difficult to refuse	7.84	0.002	(1.66 28.33)	6.54	0.005	(1.76 24.21)
One smokes because I like the taste	12.25	0.000	(5.06 29.65)	11.25	0.000	(4.59 27.58)
One smokes because it give me energy	7.84	0.105	(4.14 14.82)	7.14	0.000	(3.72 13.70)
Help me face difficulties with confidence	8.21	0.082	(3.70 18.19)	7.71	0.021	(3.44 17.27)

**=p<0.05.*

Table 3.
Logistic regression (odds ratio, 95%CI and P-value)) for the association between waterpipe tobacco use and associated risk factors amongst University of Limpopo students aged 17–43 years.

associated with using waterpipe tobacco products even after adjusting for age, gender and receiving a bursary (on Campus OR=3.8095%CI 2.59 5.57) off-campus (0.26 95%CI 0.18 0.39). Liking the taste (OR= 7.84 95%CI 1.66 28.33) and difficult to refuse (OR= 12.25 95%CI 5.06 29.65) were significant ($p<0.05$) using the waterpipe even after adjusting for age gender and receiving bursary (Liking the taste (OR= 6.54 95%CI 1.76 24.21) and difficult to refuse (OR-11.25 95%CI 4.59 27.58).

4. Discussion

This cross-sectional study aimed to investigate the prevalence of waterpipe tobacco product use and associated risk factors among University of Limpopo students aged 17–43 years. The current study confirms a high prevalence (40%) of ever waterpipe smoking and low prevalence of current (6.7%) waterpipe users. Daradka et al. [16] reported the prevalence of 24.2 and 36.04% for current and ever using waterpipe smoking, respectively, amongst University students. The prevalence of ever water smoking was almost 60.7% among Iranian medical students with the current waterpipe smoking prevalence reaching 18.7 and 51% for Iranian medical students and health science students [20]. Waterpipe smoking has become a global public health problem and requires serious attention [21].

In the current study, the prevalence of ever (40.2 vs 26.3%) and current (6.7 vs 3.0%) waterpipe user was significantly ($p<0.05$) high for boys compared with girls amongst University of Limpopo students in each group. Male participants were more likely to report current waterpipe smoking and higher frequencies than their female counterparts as reported by Salloum et al. [22]. However, the current use of waterpipe is not consistent with that of studies in Western Cape Universities, Pretoria Universities and Johannesburg as researchers reported proportion of both males and females being high for both the current and ever water pipe users in these universities [7, 13, 23–25]. An effective waterpipe tobacco control is needed to curb the spread of this dangerous epidemic among both genders in university communities.

In the current study, older age at onset (21–25 years) appeared to be significantly associated with waterpipe smoking usage compared with younger age onset (less than 20 years). Similar findings were reported in other studies [21]. These associations are suggestive and reflect more dependence on waterpipe smoking which may be reflective of social behaviour in university environments. These findings are not surprising given that the older onset of tobacco use is associated with higher nicotine dependence [26]. Furthermore, older students are more conversant with the university environment than first and second-year entering students.

Having friends who are smokers and enjoying the taste were the highest risk factors for waterpipe use among the University of Limpopo students. Similar findings were reported amongst dental students at King Saud University in Riyadh [27]. Student residences were the main factor associated with waterpipe smoking among university students in the current study. University campuses are an ideal setting to reach waterpipe tobacco users and those who may initiate this while on campus [28]. Evidence-based interventions, including tobacco-free campus policies [28] are essential to decrease the initiation and continued use of all forms of tobacco products among university students and across the lifespan [29]. There is a need to further understand factors which may motivate university students to initiate waterpipe tobacco in order to develop prevention intervention [30].

Research had generated a consistent picture of the health risks of waterpipe smoking in the past. Waterpipe smokers clearly show exposure to nicotine, toxicants and carcinogens associated with smoking-induced disease [6, 31]. Waterpipe smoking acutely decreases heart rate variability and elevates CO, plasma nicotine, blood pressure and heart rate [14]. Furthermore, waterpipe smoking can cause or accelerate the rate of pulmonary and cardiovascular complications as well as cancer [32, 33]. Children exposed to waterpipe smoking have been shown to have higher levels of carcinogenic tobacco-specific nitrosamines [34]. It is suggested that several educational and consultation courses could improve habits and the attitude of students regarding the detrimental effects and dire consequences of waterpipe usage amongst the university community. It is also suggested that implementing strict surveillance on the behaviour of students in the hostel and residential places of students, along with direct cooperation of students' families, is important in reducing, if not completely eradicating, waterpipe usage. Furthermore, the university should provide enough recreation facilities for students as they spent most of their time on campus than at home.

This study has some limitations. First, data collection was based on convenience samples, without systematic regulation of sampling factors. As such, findings may not be generalizable to a broader population, including those who have never tried waterpipe smoking. Sampling was limited to university students and did not include other non-university youth and adult sub-populations around the university. Thirdly, we did not consider health risk factors related to smoking including respiratory complications the students may have ever experienced. Fourthly, the study was cross-sectional; therefore, a change in tobacco use over several years was not examined.

A comprehensive questionnaire which covered almost all aspects of daily lives was another positive point of this survey. The findings from the current study can serve as a basis for additional research to document the public health impact of waterpipe smoking and guide regulatory efforts for waterpipe smoking control in the Limpopo Province of South Africa. Future research would generate new evidence to advance waterpipe tobacco control policies.

5. Conclusions

Our results demonstrate that waterpipe smoking was more prevalent among university male students than female students. Staying on campus or off-campus was significantly ($p<0.05$) associated with using waterpipe tobacco products. Liking the taste and difficult to refuse were possible risk factors significantly associated with waterpipe usage amongst university students. Future studies should investigate the relationship of waterpipe use and the development of chronic diseases lifestyle over time.

Acknowledgements

The authors are obligated to the administrators of the Ellisras Longitudinal Study for administration of the study project.

Funding

The study received funding from the South African National Research Foundation (Reference: RA18092336171, Grant No: 127507) and the University of Limpopo (Account number: N533) for the Ellisras Longitudinal Study is acknowledged with gratitude. Any opinions, findings and conclusions or recommendations expressed in this material are those of the authors and therefore the funding sources do not accept any liability in regard thereto.

Conflicts of interest

The authors declare no conflict of interest.

Author contributions

Conceptualization, KDM.; methodology, KDM, PJM; software, KDM.; validation, HJS formal analysis, KDM; investigation, HJS; resources, HJS, KDM; data curation, KDM, PJM writing—original draft preparation, KDM.; writing—review and editing, PJM, HJS.; visualization, KDM.; supervision, KDM.; project administration, KDM ; funding acquisition, KDM.

Author details

Kotsedi Daniel Monyeki[1]*, Hlengani James Siweya[2] and Phut Johanna Makgae[1]

1 Department of Physiology and Environmental Health, University of Limpopo, Sovenga, South Africa

2 Executive Dean of Science and Agriculture, University of Limpopo, Sovenga, South Africa

*Address all correspondence to: kotsedi.monyeki@ul.ac.za

References

[1] Combrink A, Irwin N, Naidoo K, Plagerson S, Mathee A. High prevalence of hookah smoking among secondary school students in a disadvantaged community in Johannesburg. SAMJ. 2010;**100**:297-299

[2] Fawibe AE, Shittu AO. Prevalence and characteristics of cigarette smokers among undergraduates of the University of Ilorin, Nigeria. Nigerian Journal of Clinical Practice. 2011;**14**(2):201-205. DOI: 10.4103/1119-3077.84016

[3] Rayens MK, Ickes MJ, Butler KM, Wiggins AT, Anderson DG, Ellen J. Hahn University students' perceived risk of and intention to use waterpipe tobacco. Health Education Research. 2017;**32**(4):306-317

[4] Daniels KE, Roman NV. A descriptive study of the perceptions and behaviours of waterpipe use by university students in the Western Cape, South Africa. Tobacco Induced Diseases. 2013;**11**:4-8

[5] Cobb CO, Sahmarani K, Eissenberg T, Shihadeh A. Acute toxicant exposure and cardiac autonomic dysfunction from smoking a single narghile waterpipe with tobacco and with a "healthy" tobacco-free alternative. Toxicology Letters. 2012;**215**(1):70-75

[6] Aboaziza E, Eissenberg T. Waterpipe tobacco smoking: What is the evidence that it supports nicotine/tobacco dependence? Tobacco Control. 2015;**24**(suppl. 1):i44-i53

[7] Kruger L, van Walbeek C, Vellios N. Waterpipe and Cigarette Smoking among University Students in the Western Cape, South Africa. American Journal of Health Behavior. 2016;**40**:416-424

[8] Primack BA, Sidani J, Agarwal AA, Shadel WG, Donny DC, Eissenberg TE. Prevalence of and associations with waterpipe of tobacco smoking US university. Annals of Behavioral Medicine. 2008;**36**:81-86

[9] Noonan D, Patrick ME. Factors associated with perceptions of hookah addictiveness and harmfulness among young adults. Substance Abuse. 2013;**34**:83-85

[10] Heinz AJ, Giedgowd GE, Crane NA, Veilleux JC, Conrad M, Braun AR, et al. A comprehensive examination of hookah smoking in college students: Use patterns and contexts, social norms and attitudes, harm perception, psychological correlates and co-occurring substance use. Addictive Behaviors. 2013;**38**:2751-2760

[11] Khattab A, Javid A, Ghali I, Alzaabi A, Kheder AB, Koniski ML, et al. Smoking habits in the Middle East and North: Results of the BREATHE study. Respiratory Medicine. 2012;**106**:16-24

[12] Kilic DS, Kasap MY. Survey for describing student's smoking behaviour. Procedia—Social and Behavioral Sciences. 2013;**116**:298-302

[13] Van der Merwe N, Banoobhai Y, Gqweta A, Gwala A, Masiea T, Misra M, et al. Hookah pipe smoking among health science student. SAMJ. 2013;**103**:847-849

[14] Miri-Moghaddam M, Shahrakipour M, Nasseri S, Miri-Moghaddam E. Higher prevalence of water pipe compared to cigarette smoking among medical students in Southeast Iran. Central European Journal of Public Health. 2019;**27**(3): 188-194. DOI: 10.21101/cejph.a5615

[15] Daradka H, Khabour O, Alzoubi K, Nakkash R, Eissenberg T. Tobacco and waterpipe use among university students in Saudi Arabia: Impact of tobacco sales ban. Eastern Mediterranean Health Journal. 2019;**25**(2):111-118. DOI: 10.26719/emhj.18.021

[16] Othman N, Kasem AO, Faisal A. Salih Waterpipe Smoking among University Students in Sulaimaniyah, Iraqi Kurdistan: Prevalence, attitudes, and associated factors. Tanaffos. 2017;**16**(3):225-232

[17] Mashita RJ, Themane MJ, Monyeki KD. Current smoking among rural South African children: Ellisras Longitudinal Study. BMC Paediatrics. 2011;**11**:58-66

[18] Lauer RM, Clarke WR. Childhood risk factors for high adult blood pressure: The mascatine study. Pediatrics. 1989;**84**:633-641

[19] Altman DG. Practical statistics for Medical Research. London: Chapman & Hall; 1991. pp. 32-88

[20] Sabahy AR, Divsalar K, Bahreinifar S, Marzban M, Nakhaee N. Waterpipe tobacco use among Iranian university students: Correlates and perceived reasons for use. The International Journal of Tuberculosis and Lung Disease. 2011;**15**(6):844-847

[21] Maziak W, Taleb ZB, Bahelah R, Islam F, Jaber R, Auf R, et al. The global epidemiology of waterpipe smoking. Tobacco Control. 2015;**24**(Suppl. 1):i3-i12

[22] Salloum RG, Lee JH, Mostafa A, Abu-Rmeileh NME, Hamadeh RR, Darawad MW, et al. Waterpipe tobacco smoking among University Students in Three Eastern Mediterranean Countries: Patterns, place, and price. Substance Use & Misuse. 2019;**54**(14):2275-2283. DOI: 10.1080/10826084.2019.1645177

[23] Mandil A, BinSaeed A, Ahmad S, Al-Dabbagh R, Alsaadi M, Khan M. Smoking among university students: A gender analysis. Journal of Infection and Public Health. 2010;**3**:179-187

[24] Mbatchou Ngahane BH, Luma H, Mapoure YN, Fotso ZM, Afane Ze E. Correlates of cigarette smoking among university students in Cameroon. The International Journal of Tuberculosis and Lung Disease. 2013;**17**:270-274

[25] Meysamie A, Ghaletaki R, Haghazali M, Asgari F, Rashidi A, Khalilzadeh O, et al. Pattern of tobacco use among the Iranian adult population: Results of the national survey of risk factors of non-communicable diseases. Tobacco Control. 2010;**19**:125-128

[26] Sharapova SR, Phillips E, Sirocco K, Kaminski JW, Leeb RT, Rolle I. Effects of prenatal marijuana exposure on neuropsychological outcomes in children aged 1-11 years: A systematic review. Paediatric and Perinatal Epidemiology. 2018;**32**(6):512-532. DOI: 10.1111/ppe.12505

[27] AlSwuailem AS, AlShehri MK, Al-Sadhan S. Smoking among dental students at King Saud University: Consumption patterns and risk factors. Saudi Dental Journal. 2014;**26**(3):88-95. DOI: 10.1016/j.sdentj.2014.03.003

[28] Lee YO, Bahreinifar S, Ling PM. Understanding tobacco-related attitudes among college and non-college young adult hookah and cigarette users. Journal of American College Health. 2014;**62**:10-18

[29] American College Health Association. Position statement on tobacco on college and university campuses. Journal of American College Health. 2009;**58**:291-292

[30] Martinasek M, Bryant CA. Antecedents of university students' hookah smoking intention. American Journal of Health Behavior. 2013;**37**:599-609

[31] El-Zaatari ZM, Chami HA, Zaatari GS. Health effects associated with waterpipe smoking. Tobacco Control. 2015;**24**(Suppl. 1):i31-i43

[32] Nasseri S, Gurusamy M, Jung B, Lee D, Khang G, Doods H, et al. Kinin B1 receptor antagonist BI113823 reduces acute lung injury. Critical Care Medicine. 2015;**43**(11):e499-e507

[33] Gurusamy M, Nasseri S, Lee H, Jung B, Lee D, Khang G, et al. Kinin B1 receptor antagonist BI113823 reduces allergen-induced airway inflammation and mucus secretion in mice. Pharmacological Research. 2016;**104**:132-139

[34] Kassem NOF, Daffa RM, Liles S, Jackson SR, Kassem NO, Mehta S, et al. Children's exposure to second hand and third hand smoke carcinogens and toxicants in homes of hookah smokers. Nicotine & Tobacco Research. 2014;**16**:961-975

Chapter 9

Visual Impairment and Its Associated Factors among People Living with Type-2 Diabetes Mellitus at Dessie Town Hospitals, Northeast Ethiopia, 2020

Mohammed Abdu Seid, Mengistie Diress, Yonas Akalu and Baye Dagnew Mekonnon

Abstract

Visual impairment (VI) is a functional limitation of the eye(s) that results in reduced visual acuity, visual field loss, visual distortion, perceptual difficulties, or any combination of the above. Type-2 diabetes mellitus (T2DM) is one of the common causes of VI. The current study aimed to determine the prevalence and predictors of VI in diabetes individuals. Institution-based cross-sectional study was carried out, and VI was measured using visual acuity test. We used Epi Data 3.1 and SPSS - 21for data entry and statistical analysis, respectively. To find statistically linked factors of VI, we used both binary and multivariable logistic regression. The strength of association was estimated using AOR at 95% CI. Statistical significance was declared at p less than 0.05. The present study revealed 37.58% of people have VI, which is statistically linked to age, lack of regular exercise, diabetes for >5 years, insulin treatment, and poor glycemic control. Finally, individuals with T2DM who had VI accounted for more than a third of those treated in Dessie town hospitals. Advanced age, poor frequent exercise, longer duration of diabetes, and insulin are predictors. To lower the risk of VI and visual loss, early identification of VI through screening and regular follow-up is recommended.

Keywords: visual impairment, type-2 diabetes mellitus, associated factors, Ethiopia

1. Introduction

1.1 Statement of the problem

Type-2 diabetes mellitus (T2DM) is a global metabolic disease, mainly seen in developing countries [1]. Patients with T2DM are highly prone to have cardiovascular disease, renal failure, neurological problems, and retinopathy [2, 3]. If the vision of an individual has been lost once due to diabetic retinopathy, usually it could not be restored, despite some forms that probably may be treated by complex vitreoretinal surgery [1–3].

Visually impaired people (VI) could not maintain employment, productivity, independence, their medical expense, or they may not be able to legally licensed to drive, they get difficulties in reading and fail to work inorder to obtain wages to their family and execute their social responsibilities as a whole [4, 5]. It also has been linked to falls, injury, and worsened status in spanning mental health, cognition, social function, and educational attainment [6]. People developing visual impairment(s) encounter a significant challenge. They experience major life changes, such as general health limitations or loss of nearby family member [1, 6]. They also are at higher risk of violence and abuse, which limit them from participating in and contributing to their families and societies on an equal basis with others [7].

Globally, prevalence of visual impairment increased sharply from 441.1 million [8] to 2.2 billion [4]. Of which at least 1 billion of VI could have been prevented. Among the causes of visual impairment, 1% was associated with diabetic retinopathy [9]. Diabetic retinopathy is damage to blood vessels in the retina, swelling in the central part of the retina, and abnormal blood vessels formation, which can lead to bleed or cause scarring of the retina that results in visual impairment [10].

Sub-Saharan Africa report on visual impairment figures out that the prevalence of visual impairment was 29.7% among diabetes mellitus [11]. Cataract, diabetic retinopathy, glaucoma, and maculopathy were the causes of visual impairment. Ethiopian systematic review and meta-analysis report revealed that the prevalence of diabetic retinopathy among diabetes mellitus patients was 19.48%, which is one cause of preventable visual impairment among middle-age and elderly populations [12].

In Ethiopia, no research is done on visual impairment among diabetes mellitus patients. But one previous study at the same setting found that visual disturbance was the second major chronic complication among newly diagnosed diabetes mellitus patients that was detected by clinical findings and questionnaire-based approaches. Moreover, specific associated factors for developing visual impairment had not been assessed. In parallel to rapid increment of DM, visual impairment is still public health challenge due to its chronic impacts.

Therefore, this study is designed to assess the magnitude and associated factors of long-term complication of DM, particularly vision impairments among both newly diagnosed and old type 2 diabetes mellitus patients having follow-up in Dessie town hospitals, northeastern Ethiopia, using ocular examinations and ocular tests. Since diabetes mellitus is a lifelong disease, the findings of this study will be used as input for all stakeholders such as governments, healthcare providers, people living with DM, civil society, food producers, and manufacturers and suppliers of medicines and technology. Collectively, they can make a significant contribution to halt the most serious and feared diabetes mellitus complication, (i.e., vision loss) and improve their lives as well.

1.2 Literature review

1.2.1 Definition and classification of visual impairment

Visual impairment (VI) is a functional limitation of the eye(s) due to a disorder or disease that results in reduced visual acuity, visual field loss, photophobia, diplopia, visual distortion, visual perceptual difficulties, or any combination of the above [13]. Visual impairment is also often defined as presented visual acuity of worse than either 20/40 Or 20/60 to no light perception (NLP) in either or both eyes [14].

Visual impairment can be congenital or hereditary. Other main causes of VI incude refractive error, cataract, glaucoma, corneal opacity, age-related macular degeneration, and diabetic retinopathy [4, 13, 15–17]. It is also linked to ocular infection or disease, trauma, and systemic diseases such as hyperthyroidism [18], rheumatoid arthritis, HIV/AIDS, and hypertension [19].

Visual impairment in category Inernational Classification of Disease code H54 (H54) comprises from category 0 to 9 based on presenting distance on visual acuity test and classified as low vision (mild, moderate, and severe visual impairments) and blindness [4, 20] (annex VI).

1.2.2 Pathogenesis of visual impairment due to diabetes mellitus

Chronic hyperglycemia following long-standing DM is claimed to cause visual impairment via the production of inflammatory factors, which lead to inflammation of endothelium that in turn reduces the integrity of the blood retinal barrier in diabetic eyes [21, 22]. These are attributed to decreased in the activity of nitric oxide, increased in the activity of angiotensin II, endothelin-1, and vascular endothelial growth factor (VEGF) [3]. Besides, there is slow growth of new blood vessels in the iris and trabecular meshwork, which inhibits outflow of the aqueous humor fluid that causes irreversible damage to the optic nerve, eventually leading to blindness [21]. Disruption of the blood retinal barrier is responsible for developing retinovascular diseases including diabetic retinopathy (DR). Henceforth, DR causes vascular leakage and macular edema. If timely management is not tailored, there will be reduced vision and eventually blindness [2, 23].

Diabetes-associated glucose toxicity leads to biochemical changes due to polyol pathway and activation of protein kinase C (PKC) [24]. The polyol pathway is started by the conversion of glucose to sorbitol by the aldose reductase, and then sorbitol is changed into fructose by sorbitol dehydrogenase [25]. Accumulation of sorbitol leads to osmotic changes resulting in hydropic lens fibers that degenerate lens and form sugar cataracts [26]. Both polyol pathway and PKC result in increased oxidative stress, inflammation, and vascular incompetence. Oxidative stress and inflammation cause upregulation of growth factors that play a role in the breakdown of the blood retinal barrier and development of macular edema [26, 27]. Chronic hyperglycemia also increases diacylglycerol (DAG) that leads to the activation of protein PKC. Then PKC increases vascular permeability and upregulation of retinal vascular endothelial growth factors. Diacylglycerol and PKC pathways progressively affect inflammation, neovascularization, and retinal blood flow, which ends up with DR and progressively visual impairment [27, 28].

1.2.3 Prevalence of visual impairment among type-2 diabetic mellitus patients

Pandemicity of T2DM is rising rapidly probably due to increasing obesity, reduced physical exercise as countries become more industrialized and aging of the population [6]. Between 2010 and 2030, a 20% increase DM cases in developed countries and a 69% increase in developing countries have been predicted [29]. According to WHO report, currently global prevalence of visually impaired people is estimated to be 2.2 billion. Of these, at least 1 billion visual impairment is preventable or has yet to be addressed [4].

Many studies were conducted in different countries on the prevalence of visual impairment among T2DM. VI among T2DM in Sankara Nethralaya was 4% [30], Peru 26.3% [31], China 10% [16], Jordan 17.7% [32], Turkey 16.2% [33], and Yemenian 76.5% [34].

Studies in Africa reported different magnitude of VI. The prevalence of unilateral visual impairment among DM patients was 78.25% in South Africa [35], 17.1% in Zambia [36], and 18.4% in Kumasi, Ghana [37]. In Nigerian, 24.1% of T2DM cases had visual impairment [38]. Moreover observational studies in Tunisia [39] and Cameron [40] revealed 22.2% and 22.6% prevalence of VI among DM patients, respectively.

In Ethiopia, there is no visual impairment study done among diabetes mellitus patients, but in a study at St. Paul's Hospital, visual impairment was 17.6% among all ophthalmic cases. Of this, 58.7% had low vision and 41.3% had blindness [23] and that of Dessie referral Hospital, the prevalence of visual disturbance among diabetes mellitus patients was 28.9% [41].

1.2.4 Associated factors of visual impairment among T2DM patients

Factors associated for developing visual impairment vary among different studies. A study done in China, Jordan, and Yemen revealed that visual impairment was statistically associated to patients' age, duration of diabetes, body mass index (23.4 ± 3.9), education level ($\leq$ primary education), and insulin as treatment option [16, 32, 42].

Finding from Sankara Nethralaya showed that visual impairment was higher among diabetes patients age > 60 years and low socioeconomic status [30]. In Peruvian population, hypertension, hemoglobin A1c, and use of insulin or sulfonylurase as diabetic treatment were associated to visual impairment [31]. Diabetes and visual impairment study in sub-Saharan Africa (evidence from Cameroon) revealed that factors such as age ($\geq$ 50), duration ($\geq$10 years), and hypertension were associated with severe visual impairment [11]. A study from Zambia, Turkey, and Tunisia findings indicated that age, overweight, duration of diabetes, high random blood sugar, high systolic blood pressure, and insulin as diabetic treatment were significantly associated to visual impairment [33, 36, 39].

In Arbaminch Referral Hospital, baseline age ($\geq$ 60), duration of diabetes ($\geq$6), baseline systolic BP level (>140) were significantly associated to DR [43] while in Dessie, patients' age, drug regimen, and specific medications taken were associated with diabetic complication (**Figure 1**) [41].

1.2.5 Developed conceptual framework

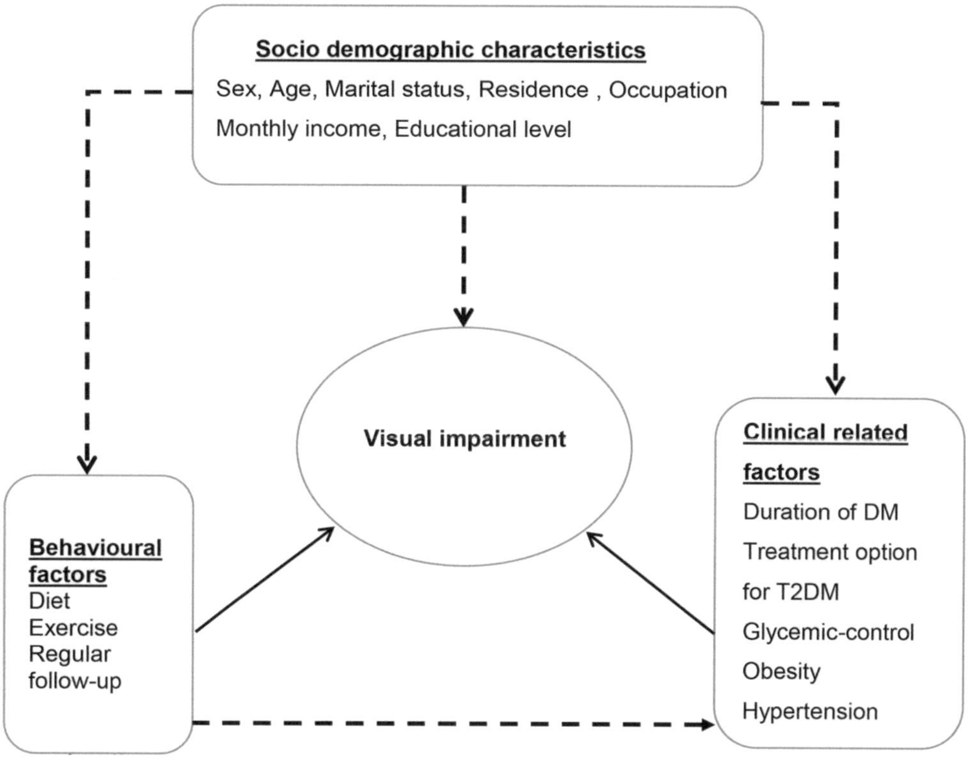

Figure 1.
Conceptual framework adapted from different literatures illustrating possible factors affecting visual impairment among people living with T2DM at Dessie, Northeast Ethiopia, 2020 [11, 16, 31, 32, 36, 39, 43].

1.3 Justification of the study

To the best of my knowledge, there was no study conducted in Ethiopia to determine the prevalence of VI and its associated factors among people living with T2DM. Vision loss is the most serious and feared outcome of DM-associated complication. After completion, this study will provide an in-depth and comprehensive information on the prevalence of VI and identify associated factors among people living with T2DM. The findings of this study will enable DM patients to implement preventive strategies and adhere to self-care management and medication to improve glycemic control and hence preventing VI by targeting associated factors. Preventive strategies include screening for DR, provision of follow-up care, and ensuring the follow-up techniques that meet the standard clinical guidelines. Making available an adequate referral mechanism allows all patients to screen and diagnose DM early so that possible ensuring eye complications are detected. Indeed, it will create an effort to develop effective health service programs and policies for better management of DM and cost-effective strategies in Ethiopian context as well as a baseline for the coming researchers and stakeholders at higher level.

2. Objectives

2.1 General objective

- The aim of the current study was to assess the prevalence of visual impairment and its associated factors among people living with T2DM at Dessie Town Hospitals, Northeast Ethiopia, 2020

2.2 Specific objectives

- To determine the prevalence of VI among people living with T2DM
- To identify associated factors of VI among people living with T2DM

3. Methods and materials

3.1 Study setting and period

This study was conducted at Dessie town hospitals (both government and private hospitals). Dessie town is located 400 km away from Addis Ababa, the capital city of Ethiopia. During the study period, there were four private and one governmental referral hospitals in Dessie town. Current report of Dessie zonal administrative office showed that these hospitals engaged in providing service for more than 3.5 million people. According to annual summative report of all diabetic clinics in Dessie town hospitals, an estimated number of 14,000 people living with T2DM were served. In each hospital, there was diabetic follow-up clinic for treatment and follow-up of people living with DM. The follow-up date in each hospital was from Monday to Friday. The actual data collection period was from February 15, to March. 152,020.

3.2 Study design

Institution-based cross-sectional study design was employed.

3.3 Source population

Source population was all people living with type-2 diabetes mellitus (both old and newly diagnosed cases) came to diabetic clinic of each hospital.

3.4 Study population

Study population was all people living with type-2 diabetes mellitus visiting diabetic clinic of each hospital during data collection period.

3.5 Eligibility criteria

3.5.1 Inclusion criteria

People living with T2DM who had follow-up and newly diagnosed T2DM patients in diabetic clinic during study period were included in the study.

3.5.2 Exclusion criteria

People living with T2DM who were seriously ill, pregnant women, and those who had HIV/AIDS, trachoma, acute eye infections (bacterial or viral), trauma to the eye, history of head injury, and history of stroke were excluded from the study.

3.6 Sample size determination and sampling technique

Sample size was determined using a single population proportion formula by considering the following assumptions:

Prevalence of visual impairment =28.9% [41], 95% confidence interval ($z\alpha/2$). and 5% margin of error (d = 0.05). Then sample size (n):

$$n = \frac{(Z\alpha/2)^2 p(1-p)}{d^2}. \tag{1}$$

$$n = (1.96)^2 \times (0.289) \times (0.711)/(0.05)^2 = 316 \tag{2}$$

Adding non-response rate of 5% yielding a final sample size of 332.

Sample size allocation.

Sample size for each hospitals was allocated by using sample size allocation formula.

$$n_j = \frac{n}{N} N_j \tag{3}$$

Where n_j = sample size for each hospitals.

n = total sample size.

Nj = total people living with type 2 diabetes in each hospitals.

N = total people living with type 2 diabetes in all hospitals.

$$\mathbf{n}_{DRH} = \frac{332}{14000} * 10210 = 242 \tag{4}$$

$$\mathbf{n}_{SRH} = \frac{332}{14000} * 1440 = 34 \tag{5}$$

$$\mathbf{n}_{ERH} = \frac{332}{14000} * 1250 = 30 \tag{6}$$

$$\mathbf{n}_{BRH} = \frac{332}{14000} * 1100 = 26 \tag{7}$$

Where DRH = Dessie Referral Hospital, SRH=Selam General Hospital, ESH = Ethio General Hospital and BGH=Bati General Hospital (**Figure 2**).

In this study, Dessie Referral Hospital and all private hospitals were included and simple random sampling technique using lottery methods was applied to recruit study participants from those of type 2 DM cases who came to the clinic for follow-up and newly diagnosed T2DM patients during study period.

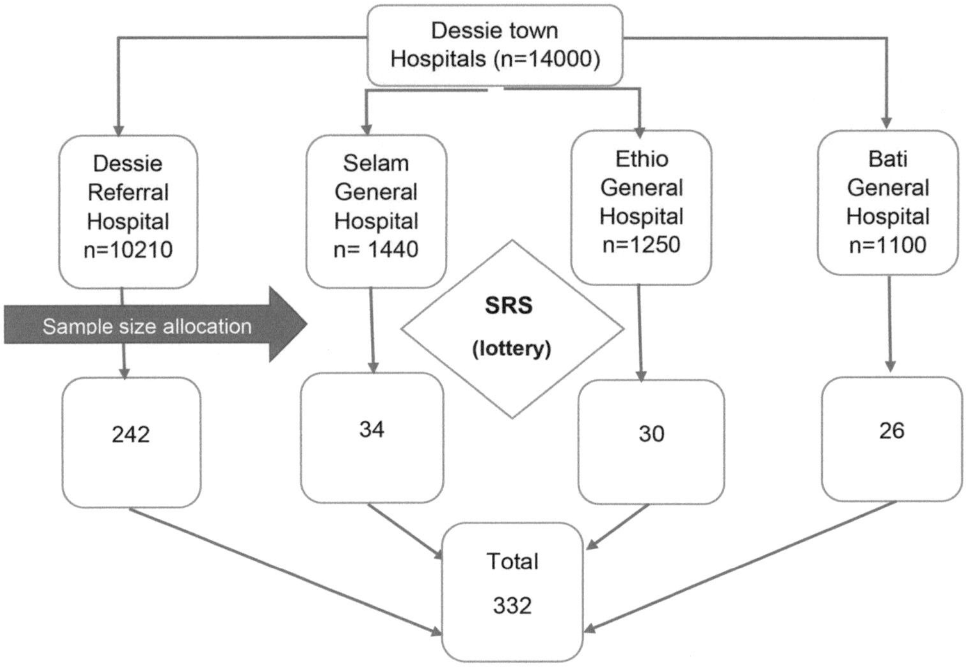

Figure 2.
Diagrammatic representation of sampling procedure for T2DM at Dessie town Hospitals, Northeast Ethiopia, 2020.

3.7 Study variables

3.7.1 Dependent variable

- Visual impairment

3.7.2 Independent variables

- **Sociodemographic variables**: Age in years, sex, monthly income, marital status, and educational level
- **Behavioral variables:** Diet, exercise, and diabetic regular follow-up to T2DM
- **Clinical-related variables**: Glycemic control, plasma glucose level, duration of DM, comorbidities (hypertension and obesity), and treatment option for people living with type 2 diabetes mellitus.

3.8 Operational definitions

Visual impairment: Is any loss or abnormality in an anatomical structure or a physiological or psychological function [13]. It is presenting visual acuity of worse than either 20/40 0r 20/60 to no light perception (NLP) in either or both eyes, which includes both low vision and blindness [44].

Low vision: Even with corrective lenses, it is inability to clearly see at a distance of 6 meters (20 feet) that individuals with normal vision can clearly see at a distance of 12 meters (40 feet) or visual acuity between 6/12 and 3/60. Low vision includes mild visual impairment (VA between 6/12 and 6/18), "moderate visual impairment (VA between 6/18 and 6/60)" and "severe visual impairment (VA between 6/60 and 3/60)" from all causes [4].

Blindness: Inability to read the largest letter on a vision chart at a distance of 3 meters (10 feet) or visual acuity was worse than 3/60 [45].

Visual acuity/VA: Simple, noninvasive measure of the visual system's ability to discriminate two high-contrast points in space. It is usually taken at a distance of 6 m or 20 feet [9]. It is expressed in terms of A/B, where A: distance b/n observer and letters and B: expected distance that the health eye can observe.

Obesity: A BMI of ≥ 30 kg/m^2 is considered obese. Class 1 obesity (BMI: 30–34.9 kg/m^2) is one of the most common subtypes. Obesity class 2 (BMI 35–39.9 kg/m^2), extreme obesity or morbid obesity (BMI 40 kg/m^2) is classified as class 3 (BMI 40 kg/m^2) [46].

Exercise: Exercising for less than 150 minutes per 3–5 days/week is regarded poor, while exercising for more than 150 minutes per 3–5 days per week is considered good [47].

3.9 Data collection procedures and tools

We used semistructured interviewer-administered questionnaire, tape meter, and weight balance to collect data. Type of diabetes already diagnosed by physician and their ID list were used to select study participants. After obtaining consent, weight, height, and blood pressure were taken. Then they were scheduled for eye examination at the eye clinic of the same institution and had additional benefits of individualized counseling, care, and referral depending on the ocular findings. At the eye clinic, each patient had visual acuity assessment with illuminated Snellen's chart for each eye at 6 m. Training was given by principal investigator about the objective of study, data collection techniques, and ethical issues had been given to four data collectors who were BSc ophthalmic nurses and clinical nurses and one supervisor prior to actual data collection. Pre-test was applied on 17 patients in Borumeda General Hospital for evaluation of consistency, approachability, and feasibility of the questionnaire. Information obtained was strictly kept confidential.

3.9.1 Ophthalmic examination

Ophthalmic examination was performed by ophthalmic nurse and ophthalmologist. Careful ocular history, inspection, and examination of the eye using slit-lamp and dilated fundus examination were conducted. Visual acuity (using snellen chart), macular degeneration (ophthalmoscope), intraocular pressure (using tonometry), and history of night blindness for vitamin A deficiency were taken.

3.9.2 Snellen chart for visual acuity test

Visual acuity is measured by taking 6 m notation. Visual acuity was performed in a properly illuminated quiet room, using Snellen chart at 6 m to discriminate different letters. Each eye was tested separately, and the procedure was repeated, then the best average was taken. The person who could identify the letters of the size 6 at 6 m (20 at

20 feet) was said to have normal vision. The numerator expresses the distance between the observer and the letters while the denominator expresses the distance at which the letter could be distinguished by the normal eye.

3.10 Data quality control

Data quality assurance was maintained starting from design. The questionnaire was first prepared in English and then translated from English to Amharic (local language) and retranslated to Amharic by another expert to ensure understanding of the items for the participants and its consistency. Pre-test was done on 17 people living with T2DM at Borumeda Hospital. Training was given for data collectors and supervisor on the data collection tool and ethical issues during data collection.

3.11 Data processing and statistical analysis

After completing the data collection process, data were entered into Epi data-3.1 by data entry clerk, then exported into SPSS version 22 for analysis. Data completeness, consistency, and outliers were checked. Continues data were described by median and inter-quartile range while frequency with percent was used to describe the results of categorical variables. Then results were presented using tabulation, graph, and charts. Uni-variable analysis was used to describe independent variables, and bi-variable binary logistic regression analysis was performed to select potential candidate variables for the final model with cutoff point of p value $\leq$0.25 [48]. Model fitness was checked by Hosmer and Lemeshow goodness of fit test. Multivariable binary logistic regression analysis was done to identify significant factors of visual impairment. Adjusted odds ratio with 95% CI was computed to show significant factors. In the final model, variables with a p value $\leq$0.05 were considered as statistically significant.

4. Ethical consideration

The institutional review board (IRB) of the University of Gondar, College of Medicine and Health Sciences, granted ethical approval with reference number 1839/02/2020. Prior to data collection, Dessie Town Hospitals provided an official authorization letter. After describing the goal of the study to each participant, they signed a written informed consent form. Participants had full mandate to participate or to refuse even to withdraw at any time they want from the study. The information obtained was kept confidential.

5. Dissemination plan of results

Electronic copy of the thesis will be published by University of Gondar for online access. We also plan to disseminate the result of this study as a copy of the document to Dessie town private hospitals and Dessie Refferal Hospital. Attempts will be made to present the findings at various scientific conferences, workshops, and meetings. In addition, an effort will be made to publish the findings in a peer-reviewed scientific journal.

6. Results

6.1 Sociodemographic characteristics of participants

Out of the total of 332 study participants, 322 have participated in the study yielding a response rate of 97%. The median age of participants was 52 years (IQR: 45–60 years) ranging from 24 to 87 years. One-hundred seventy and five (54.3%) study participants were male giving female-to-male ratio of 1: 1.18. Two hundred and twelve (65.8%) individuals were Islamic religion followers. Seventy-three (22.7%) participants were unable to read and write. One-hundred and fifteen people (35.7%) worked for a private company, 291 (90.4%) were married, and 249 (77.3%) lived in a town. The median monthly income of the participants' households was 3570 ETB (IQR: 2000–5195, Min = 800, Max = 9600ETB) (**Table 1**).

Variables	Categories	Frequency	Percent
Age in years	20–40	37	11.5
	41–59	189	58.7
	60–87	96	29.8
Sex	Male	175	54.3
	Female	147	45.7
Religion	Muslim	212	65.8
	Orthodox	103	32
	Others*	7	2.2
Marital status	Never married	31	9.6
	Married	291	90.4
Residence	Urban	249	77.3
	Rural	73	22.7
Educational level	Unable to read and write	73	22.7
	Primary	84	26.1
	Secondary	79	24.5
	Diploma and above	86	26.7
Occupation	Government workers	70	21.8
	Private workers **	115	35.7
	Farmer	37	11.5
	House wife	60	18.6
	Others***	40	12.4

Other: protestant and catholic, Private worker**: construction, daily laborer, driver, mechanic, merchant, Others***: jobless, pensioner.*

Table 1.
Sociodemographic characteristics of people living with T2DM at Dessie town Hospitals, Northeast Ethiopia, 2020 (n = 322).

6.2 Type-2 DM and vision-related characteristics of participants

Forty-six (14.3%) people living with T2DM had trouble in adjusting light while entering from bright to dim light. One-hundred and seventy three (53.7%) of DM patients had duration 5 years and less since diagnosis while 24 (7.5%) were new cases. Of all participants, two-hundred and sixty-four (82.0%) T2DM patients had regular follow-up in clinics. One-hundred and ninety nine (61.8%) of participants had poor or inadequate physical exercise. In 201 (62.4%) T2DM patients, the treatment option for DM was oral hypoglycemic agent without insulin. Thirty-seven (11.5%) participants were obese (BMI: median = 34.8, IQR: (23.1–27.65) and 98 (30.4%) individuals had co-morbid hypertension. Respondents had a median with IQR of baseline random plasma glucose (311, (260–396)) and fasting plasma glucose (160, (140–208)), respectively. One-hundred and eighty-seven (58.1%) participants had poor glycemic control (**Table 2**).

Variables	Categories	Frequency	Percent
Have trouble in adjusting light (night blindness)	Yes	46	14.3
	No	276	85.7
Regular follow-up	Yes	264	82
	No	58	18
Duration of diabetes (in years)	Newly diagnosed	24	7.5
	≤5 years	173	53.7
	>5 up to 24 years	125	25.8
Treatment (n = 296)	OHA without insulin	201	67.9
	Both of OHA and insulin	73	24.7
	Insulin only	22	7.4
Regular exercise	Good*	123	38.2
	Poor*	199	61.8
BMI (kg/m^2)	Underweight	5	1.5
	Normal	159	49.4
	Overweight	121	37.6
	Obese	37	11.5
Comorbid hypertension	Yes	98	30.4
	No	224	69.6
Glycemic control	<152 mg/dl (good)	135	41.9
	≥152 mg/dl (poor)	187	58.1

OHA: oral hypoglycemic agents, Good: doing exercise every other day ≥30 min/day, Poor*: do not doing exercise at all or doing exercise <30 min/day.*

Table 2.
Factors related to diabetes mellitus and vision-related characteristics of participants at Dessie town Hospitals, Northeast Ethiopia, 2020 (n = 322).

6.3 Prevalence of visual impairment among people living with T2DM

In the current study, the prevalence of visual impairment was 37.58% [95% CI: 32.3–42.9] with mean ± SEM (0.38 ± 0.027) (**Figure 3**).

Fifty-eight (18.0%) participants with visual impairments were in the moderate visual impairment category. Among the overall prevalence of visual impairment, 43 (13.4%) had bilateral vision impairment and 78(24.2%) had monocular vision impairment out of total participants. Of all visually impaired T2DM, 107 (33.2%) and 14 (4.4%) had low vision and blindness, respectively (**Table 3**) (**Figure 3**).

Visual impairment among people living with T2DM increases with age. Among over all T2DM patients participated in this study, three (0.93%) participants aged 20–39 years, 62 (19.25%), individuals aged 40–59 years, and 56 (17.39%) participants aged 60–87 years were visually impaired (**Figure 4**).

Visual impairment category		Frequency	Percent
<6/12–6/18	**Bilateral mild VI**	**28**	**23.1**
<6/18–6/60	Bilateral moderate VI	10	8.3
<6/60–3/60	Bilateral severe VI	1	0.8
<3/60-NLP	Bilateral blindness	4	3.3
<6/12–6/18, other eye 6/6–6/12	Monocular mild VI	0	0.0
<6/18–6/60, other eye 6/6–6/18	Monocular moderate VI	48	39.7
<6/60–3/60, other eye 6/6–6/60	Monocular severe VI	20	16.5
<3/60-NLP, other eye 6/6–3/60	Monocular blindness	10	8.3
Total		121	100

Note: NLP-no light perception, VI-visual impairment.

Table 3.
Forms of visual impairment categories among people living with T2DM at Dessie town Hospitals, Northeast Ethiopia, 2020, (n = 322).

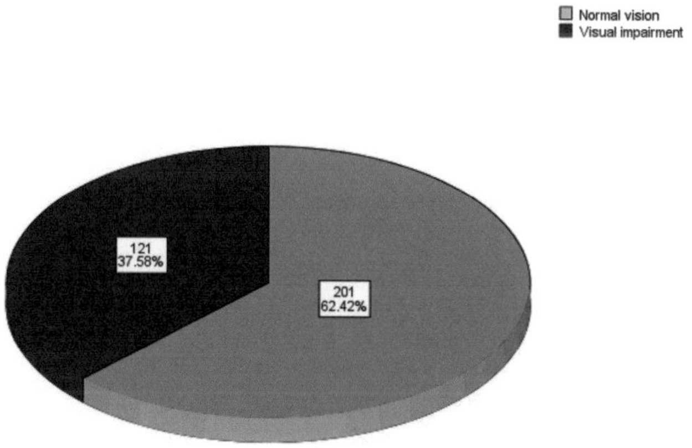

Figure 3.
Pie chart showing prevalence of visual impairment among people living with T2DM at Dessie town Hospitals, Northeast Ethiopia, 2020 (n = 322).

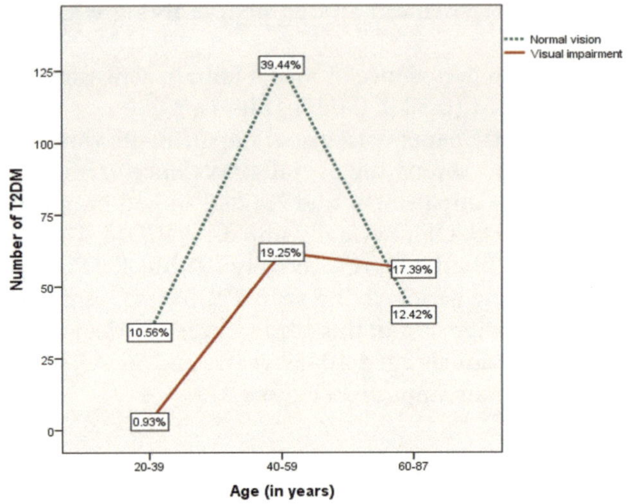

Figure 4.
Distribution of visual impairment among different age groups of people living with T2DM at Dessie town Hospitals, Northeast Ethiopia, 2020 (n = 322).

In T2DM patients, visual impairment increases with duration of diabetes. Among all T2DM participants, 1 (0.31%) new T2DM cases, 42 (13.04%) participants with 5 years and below duration, and 78 (24.22%) individuals with >5 up to 24 years of duration were visually impaired (**Figure** 5).

6.4 Associated factors of VI among patients living with T2DM

Age, sex, marital status, educational level, occupation, residence, regular exercise, duration of DM, treatment option, baseline random plasma glucose, hypertension,

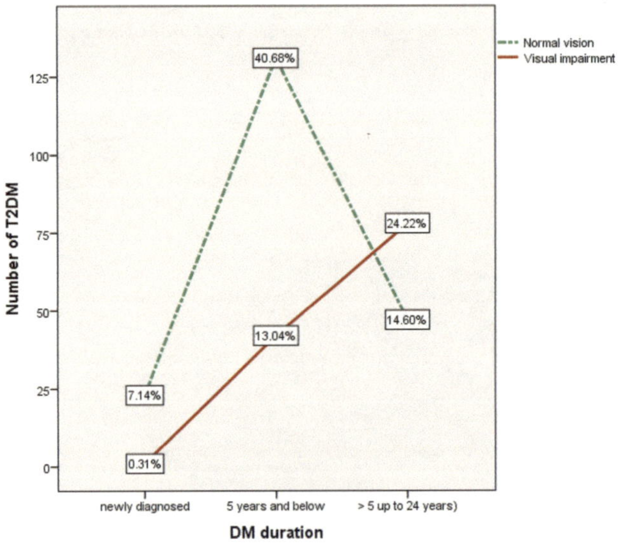

Figure 5.
Magnitude of VI across duration of people living with T2DM at Dessie town Hospitals, Northeast Ethiopia, 2020 (n = 322).

and glycemic control were candidates for final model. In multivariable analysis age, poor regular exercise, duration of diabetes, insulin treatment, and poor glycemic control were statistically significant with visual impairment.

The odds of having visual impairment for each age increase of a unit (a year) were 1.06 times (AOR: 1.06, 95% CI: 1.02, 1.09). Participants who relied on insulin were 14 times (AOR = 14.05, 95% CI: 2.72, 72.35) more likely to get visual impairment than those who used treatment options without insulin. The odds of having visual impairment in diabetes mellitus who had poor physical exercise were 2.91 times (AOR = 2.91,

Variables	Categories	VI		COR (95% CI)	AOR(95% CI)
		No	Yes		
Sex	Male	119	56	1	1
	Female	82	65	1.68 (1.06, 2.65)	1.29(0.56, 2.96)
Marital status	Unmarried	27	4	1	
	Married	174	117	4.54(1.54, 13.31)	1.25(0.30, 5.11)
Education	Unable to read and write	32	41	1	1
	Primary (1–8)	52	32	0.48 (0.25, 0.90)	0.92 (0.33 2.50)
	Secondary	51	28	0.43 (0.22, 0.82)	1.11 (0.37, 3.29)
	Diploma and above	66	20	0.23 (0.12, 0.46)	0.67 (0.20, 2.23)
Occupation	Government worker	52	18	1	1
	Private worker	81	34	1.21 (0.62, 2.36)	0.80 (0.34, 1.88)
	Farmer	23	14	1.75 (0.74, 4.12)	0.35(0.10, 1.17)
	House wife	26	34	3.77 (1.80, 7.92)	1.54 (0.59, 4.00)
	Other	19	21	3.19 (1.40, 7.25)	1.33(0.42, 4.17)
Residence	Urban	166	83	1	
	Rural	35	38	2.17(1.27, 3.68)	1.85(0.71, 4.80)
Regular-	Good	94	29	1	
exercise	Poor	107	92	2.78(1.68, 4.59)	2.91(1.47, 5.76)**
Duration of diabetes	≤5 years	154	43	1	
	>5–24 years	47	78	28.59(3.68, 221.75)	2.42(1.24, 4.73)**
Treatment	OHA without insulin	140	61	1	
	Both of OHA and insulin	34	39	2.63(1.52, 4.56)	1.45(0.71, 2.97)
	Insulin only	2	20	22.95(5.20, 101.25)	14.05(2.72, 72.35)**
Hypertension	Yes	51	47	1.86(1.15, 3.03)	1.26(0.65, 2.44)
	No	150	74	1	
Glycemic-	<152 (good)	94	41	1	
control(FPG)	≥152 (poor)	107	80	1.71(1.07, 2.73)	2.17(1.13, 4.14)*

*Note: OHA: oral hypoglycemic agent, * significant ($p < 0.05$), ** significant ($p < 0.01$), *** significant ($p < 0.001$), 1 - reference, Hosmer - Lemeshow goodness-of-fit ($p = 0.781$), no multicollinearity (VIF < 10).*

Table 4.
Multivariable binary logistic regression analysis for associated factors of visual impairment among people living with T2DM at Dessie town Hospitals, Northeast Ethiopia, 2020 (n = 322).

95% CI: 1.47, 5.76) more likely than those who were good in physical exercise. People living with T2DM with duration of more than 5 years were 2.42 times (AOR: 2.42, 95% CI: 1.24, 4.73) more likely to acquire visual impairment than those with duration of 5 years and lower. Those who had poor glycemic control were 2.17 times (AOR: 2.17, 95% CI: 1.13, 4.14) more likely to develop visual impairment in contrary to good glycemic control (**Table 4**).

7. Discussion

Despite the wide range of effects of T2DM on vision, no thorough study has been undertaken in Ethiopia to describe visual impairment and the factors that influence it among persons with T2DM. The goal of this study was to find out how common visual impairment is among persons with T2DM and what factors contribute to it in Dessie town Hospitals in Northeast Ethiopia.

At Dessie town Hospitals, the prevalence of visual impairment among people with T2DM was 37.58% (95% CI: 32.3–42.9) in the current study. This figure is greater than the 28.9% found in a prior study at Dessie Referral Hospital [41]. This disparity is likely owing to previous researchers' study designs, which included a review of patient records as a source of data, a different study population (only newly diagnosed DM), and visual disturbance was recognized using clinical findings and questionnaire-based procedures (where visual acuity test was not applied). Furthermore, the current study's prevalence of visual impairment is higher than other studies in Nigeria (24.1%) [49], Tunisia (22.2%) [39], and Cameron (29.7%). [11] Kumasi, Ghana (18.4%) [37], Zambia (17.1%) [36], Turkey (13.5%) [33], Peru (40.2%) [31], Jordan (17.7%) [32], Hengli, Southern China (10%) [44], and Sankara Nethralaya (4.1%) [30]. This disparity is most likely related to disparities in case definition, technique used, socioeconomic status, and the quality of chronic disease care services provided. The cutoff limit for VI in this investigation was VA 6/12, whereas VA 6/18 was used in the previous trials. Those investigations, unlike the current one, used the better eye's presenting visual acuity to define visual impairment. Furthermore, their research was conducted at the community level, where there was a chance of screening normal-sighted people. However, Our study was conducted in a hospital setting, and the majority of the patients had a known diabetes problem, which could lead to an increase in the prevalence of visual impairment.

In the Nigerian study, voluntary sampling and a lower sample size were used. Purposive sampling was utilized in Tunisia, which introduced bias, and both investigations defined visual impairment using the better eye presenting visual acuity. When one eye was visually impaired but the other was not, they judged it to be no vision impairment, which understates the extent of visual impairment when compared with the current study, which takes either eye's visual acuity into account.

This study found a lower rate of unilateral vision impairment than those conducted in Yemen (76.5% [34] and South Africa (78.25%) [35]. This disparity could be attributable to changes in case definitions for vision impairment and sample sizes. In the study conducted in South Africa, study participants were T2DM aged 40, with a cutoff point of VA between 6/9.5 and 6/18, which was defined as a visual impairment, whereas in Yemen, a large sample size was used, with all conditions overestimated or the possibility of adding additional visually impaired cases.

In the current study, visual impairment was significantly associated with advanced age, inadequate regular exercise, diabetes duration, insulin, and poor glycemic management.

For each unit (a year) increase in age, the likelihood of experiencing visual impairment increased by 1.06 times. A study in Tunisia [39], Southern China [16], and Sankara Nethralaya found comparable results [30]. Possible explanations include reduced activity, loss of muscle mass, and weight gain, which cause fatty cells to become more insulin resistant, resulting in hyperglycemia. Due to heart insufficiency, advanced age also increases the risk of macrovascular events [50].

The odds of having visual impairment in diabetes mellitus who had poor physical exercise were 2.91 times more likely than those who were good in physical exercise. This might be due to exercise that can promote an increase in the bioavailability of nitric oxide (NO), which decreases blood pressure, postexercise can increase in glycolipid uptake and utilization, which improves glucose homeostasis, insulin sensitivity and maintaining glycemic level [51–53], optimized body mass index, and modulated DNA methylation [54].

Participants with duration of diabetes of above 5 years were 2.42 times more likely to get visual impairment as compared with those with type 2 diabetes with duration of 5 years and below. This finding is in line with Zambia [36], Yemen [42], Peru [31], and China [16]. Possible reason might be long duration of diabetes has lower adherence [55], hall marker for long-term exposure to hyperglycemia [56], and potential increase risk of macrovascular and microvascular events and death [50]. Moreover, long duration linked to a reduction in insulin secretion or excessive insulin resistance in T2DM patients [24].

Diabetes mellitus patients who were managed by insulin only were 14 times more likely to have visual impairment than diabetes patients who are managed without insulin. This is consistence with study in Zambia [36], Turkey [33], Peru [31], Jordan [32]. and Sankara Nethralaya [28]. The reason is probably linked to the use of insulin alone that reflects less adherence [55] resulting in deterioration in kidney function, decline in β-cell function, or increase in insulin resistance over time [57], which in turn is associated with poor plasma glucose control and higher risk of severe diabetes.

The odds of being visually impaired were two times higher in poor glycemic control in contrary to good glycemic control, which is in line with study in Peruvians [31]. The possible reason might be poor glycemic control or persistent hyperglycemia damages retinal vasculature via activation of a pro-inflammatory mediators such as tumor necrotic factor (TNF)-2, interleukin-6, interleukin-1b, angiotensin II, endothelin-1, and vascular endothelial growth factor (VEGF) that could alter retinal blood barrier and lead to retinal vessel leakage causing macular edema and nerve scaring, which result in retinal detachment and sudden vision loss.

8. Conclusion

The prevalence of VI in Dessie town hospitals accounts for more than a third of patients living with type-2 DM implied that was a significant public health problem. Older age, poor regular exercise, duration of diabetes, insulin treatment, and poor glycemic control were statistically significant with visual impairment. Regular diabetes follow-up and visual screening for all type-2 DM should be done at older age group patients and for those having longer duration of diabetes, which can reduce visual morbidity and vision loss. Type-2 DM patients should control glycemic level by taking medications and through adequate and regular physical exercise.

The findings of this study are essential for visual health program planners that barriers other than economic constraints are present, which prevent adoption of desired behaviors. Public health policies with educational programs and promotion of DR screening of all T2DM are needed and timely management of DR that greatly reduces the incidence of visual impairment due to diabetes. Thus integrated effort should be in place to reduce the risk of visual impairment, manage the disease progression, and prevent vision loss as a bad consequences.

9. Strength and limitations of the study

9.1 Strength

This study gave a minute picture of the problem (visual impairment) among T2DM patients in Ethiopia and made easy to understand which factors were more important to visual impairment and vision loss as a bad consequence.

9.2 Limitations

Since the study was cross-sectional, it could not show cause-effect relationship. Recall bias was also an expected limitation. Categorization of visual impairment was based on presenting, not corrected visual acuity. HbA1c was not measured due to clients' financial issue so that physicians ordered fast plasma glucose instead of HbA1c. The HbA1C test is a reliable blood test that provides information about a person's average levels of blood glucose over the past 3 months. However, the fasting plasma glucose shows only point in time result of the diabetic patients.

10. Recommendation

- Ministry of health should develop effective and efficient health programs, policies, and strategies for preventive, curative, and rehabilitative service specific to diabetics

- Health facilities should have an adequate referral mechanism that allows all patients to screen and diagnose diabetes mellitus early through screening and regular follow-up so that it can detect possible eye complications.

- People living with T2DM should adopt standardized management protocol such as diet, physical activities, and medications to live long and prevent potential complication.

- Researchers should conduct further observational (like cohort) study.

Author details

Mohammed Abdu Seid[1]*, Mengistie Diress[2], Yonas Akalu[2] and
Baye Dagnew Mekonnon[2]

1 Unit of Human Physiology, Department of Biomedical sciences, Debre Tabor University, Debre Tabor, Ethiopia

2 Department of Human Physiology, College of Medicine and Health Sciences, University of Gondar, Gondar, Ethiopia

*Address all correspondence to: mameabdu54@gmail.com

References

[1] World Health Organisation. Global report on diabetes mellitus. 2018;35-43. [Available from]: http://www.who.int

[2] Sayin N, Kara N, Pekel G. Ocular complications of diabetes mellitus. World Journal of Disbetes [Internet]. 2015;**6**(1):92-108. Available from: http://www.wjgnet.com/esps/helpdesk.aspx

[3] Brownlee M. The pathobiology of diabetic complications: A unifying mechanism. Diabetes. 2005;**54**(6): 1615-25

[4] WHO team. World Report on Vision. 2019;5-29. Available from: http://apps.who.int/iris

[5] Eckert KA, Carter MJ, Lansingh VC, Wilson DA, João M, Frick KD, et al. A simple method for estimating the economic cost of productivity loss due to blindness and moderate to severe visual impairment. Ophthalmic Epidemiol [Internet]. 2015;22(5):349–355. Available from: http://www.tandfonline.com/loi/iope20%0AA

[6] Fauci AS, Kasper DL, Lango DL, et al. Harrison's: Principles of internal medicine. [Internet]. In: The British Journal of Psychiatry. 20th ed. Vol. Vol. 112. New York, NY, USA: McGraw-Hill; 2018. pp. 211-212. Available from: www.accessmedicine.com/harrisons

[7] Kvam MH. Experiences of Childhood Sexual Abuse among Visually Impaired Adults in Norway: Prevalence and Characteristics. Sex Abus [Internet]. 2005;**99**(1):1-24. Available from: http://www.afb.org/jvib/jvib990102.asp

[8] Bourne RRA, Flaxman SR, Braithwaite T, Cicinelli MV, Das A, Jonas JB. et al. Magnitude, temporal trends, and projections of the global prevalence of blindness and distance and near vision impairment. Lancet Glob Heal [Internet]. 2017;**17**:1-10. DOI: 10.1016/S2214-109X(17)30293-0

[9] WHO. Global data on visual impairments. 2010;3–6. Available from: www.who.int

[10] Vislisel J, Oetting T. Diabetic retinopathy: Eye RoundsOrg. 2010; (Frank 2004):1-7

[11] Jingi AM, Nansseu JRN, Noubiap JJN, Bilong Y, Ellong A. Diabetes and visual impairment in sub-Saharan Africa. Journal of Diabetes and Metabolic Disorders. 2015;**14**(21):1-8

[12] Fite RO, Lake EA, Hanfore LK. Diabetic retinopathy in Ethiopia: A systematic review and meta-analysis. Diabetes & Metabolic Syndrome. Clinical Research & Reviews Diabetic retinopathy in Ethiopia : A systematic review and. Metab Syndr Clin Res Rev [Internet]. 2019;**13**(3):1885-1891. DOI: 10.1016/j.dsx.2019.04.016

[13] Fraser Freeman K, Cole P RG, Eleanor Faye OE, Freeman PB, Gregory Goodrich OL, Stelmack JA, et al. Optometric clinical practice guideline care of the patient with visual impairment. American Optometric Association. 2007;(10):6-8

[14] Maberley DAL, Hollands H, Chuo J, Tam G. The prevalence of low vision and blindness in Canada. Eye. 2006;**10**(20): 341-346

[15] Flaxman SR, Bourne RRA, Resnikoff S, Ackland P, Braithwaite T, Cicinelli MV, et al. Global causes of blindness and distance vision impairment: A systematic review and meta-analysis. Lancet Global Health

[Internet]. 2017;**5**(12):1221-1234. DOI: 10.1016/S2214-109X(17)30393-5

[16] Cui Y, Zhang L, Zhang M, Yang X, Zhang L, Kuang J. Prevalence and causes of low vision and blindness in a Chinese population with type 2 diabetes. Scientific Reports [Internet]. 2017; 7(Aug):1-9. DOI: 10.1038/s41598-017-11365-z

[17] WHO. Global initiative for the elimination of avoidable blindness. Vis 2020,the right to sight (2006–11). 2007

[18] Pinazo-durán MD, Zanón-moreno V, García-medina JJ, Arévalo JF, Gallego-pinazo R, Nucci C. Eclectic ocular comorbidities and systemic diseases with eye involvement. Biomed Research International [Internet]. 2016;16:1-7. Available from: http://www.hindawi.com

[19] Lenake M, Sa F, Registrar S. The eye in systemic disease. South African Family Practice. 2014;**56**(1):8-14

[20] Minor M. Ratified by WHO-FIC Network at the annual meeting in Tunis. 2009;**1**(January 2008): 41

[21] Gardner T, Davila J. The neurovascular unit and the pathophysiologic basis of diabetic retinopathy. Graefe's Archive for Clinical and Experimental Ophthalmology [Internet]. 2016;(July): 1-6. DOI: 10.1007/s00417-016-3548-y

[22] Rangasamy S, Mcguire PG, Das A. Review article diabetic retinopathy and inflammation: Novel therapeutic targets. Middle East African Journal of Ophthalmology [Internet]. 2012;**19**(1): 52-59. Available from: http://www.meajo.org

[23] Cherinet FM, Tekalign SY, Anbesse DH, Bizuneh ZY. Prevalence and associated factors of low vision and blindness among patients attending St. Paul's Hospital Millennium Medical College, Addis Ababa, Ethiopia. BMC Ophthalmology [Internet]. 2018;**18**(1): 10-12. DOI: 10.1186/s12886-018-0899-7

[24] Haghighatpanah M, Sasan A, Nejad M, Haghighatpanah M, Thunga G. Osong public health and research perspectives factors that correlate with poor glycemic control in type 2 diabetes mellitus patients with complications. Osong Public Health and Research Perspectives. 2018;**9**(4):167-174

[25] Ola MS, Nawaz MI, Siddiquei MM, Al-amro S, El-asrar AMA. Diabetes and its complications recent advances in understanding the biochemical and molecular mechanism of diabetic retinopathy. Journal of Diabetes and its Complications [Internet]. 2012;**26**(1): 56-64. DOI: 10.1016/j.jdiacomp.2011.11.004

[26] Ho TW, A. MK, John H. Aldose reductase, oxidative stress, and diabetic mellitus. Frontiers in Pharmacology. 2012;**3**(May):1-8

[27] Mathebula SD. Biochemical changes in diabetic retinopathy triggered by hyperglycaemia: A review. Afr Vis Heal [Internet]. 2018;**77**(April):3-5. Available from: https://www.researchgate.net/publication/324704012

[28] Safi SZ, Qvist R, Kumar S, Batumalaie K, Shah I, Ismail B. Molecular mechanisms of diabetic retinopathy, general preventive strategies, and novel therapeutic targets. BioMed Research International [Internet]. 2014;**2014**(1):5-19. DOI: 10.1155/2014/801269

[29] Ola MS, Nawaz MI, Siddiquei MM, Al-amro S, El-asrar AMA. Diabetes and Its Complications Recent advances in understanding the biochemical and molecular mechanism of diabetic retinopathy. J Diabetes Complications

[Internet]. 2012;**26**(1):56-64. DOI: 10.1016/j.jdiacomp.2011.11.004

[30] Sankara M, Diabetic N. Prevalence of Visual Impairment and Associated. Middle East African Journal of Ophthalmology. 2012;**19**(8):129-135

[31] Villena JE, Yoshiyama CA, Sánchez JE, Hilario NL, Merin LM. Prevalence of diabetic retinopathy in Peruvian patients with type 2 diabetes. Revista Panamericana de Salud Pública. 2011;**30**(5):408-414

[32] Ajlouni KM. Prevalence of blindness and visual impairment among Jordanian diabetics. European Journal of Ophthalmology [Internet]. 2005;**15**(1):62–68. Available from: mahaamr@hotmail.com

[33] Idil A, Caliskan D, Ocaktan E. The prevalence of blindness and low vision in older onset diabetes mellitus and associated factors: A community-based study. European Journal of Ophthalmology [Internet]. 2004;**14**(4): 298–305. Available from: caliskan@medicine.ankara.edu.tr

[34] Bamashmus MA, Gunaid AA, Khandekar RB. Diabetic retinopathy , visual impairment and ocular status among patients with diabetes mellitus in Yemen : A hospital-based study. Indian Journal of Ophthalmology. 2009;**57** (December):293-298

[35] Mabaso RG, Oduntan OA. Prevalence and causes of visual impairment and blindness among adults with diabetes mellitus aged 40 years at government health facilities in the Mopani District, South Africa. 2014; **73**(1):8-15. ISSN 0378-9411 9 [Internet]. Available from: mabaso@mweb.co.za/ oduntanoa@ukzn.ac.za

[36] Lewis AD, Hogg RE, Chandran M, Musonda L, North L, Chakravarthy U, et al. Prevalence of diabetic retinopathy and visual impairment in patients with diabetes mellitus in Zambia. Eye [Internet]. 2018;**32**(1):1201-1208. DOI: 10.1038/s41433-018-0055-x

[37] Lartey SY, Aikins AK. Visual impairment amongst adult diabetics attending a tertiary outpatient clinic, Kumasi, Ghana. Ghana Medical Journal [Internet]. 2018;**52**(2):84-87. DOI: 10.4314/gmj.v52i2.4

[38] Kyari F, Tafida A, Sivasubramaniam S, Murthy GVS, Peto T. Prevalence and risk factors for diabetes and diabetic retinopathy: Results from the Nigeria national blindness and visual impairment survey. BMC Public Health [Internet]. 2014; **14**(1):1-12. Available from: http://www.biomedcentral.com/1471-2458/14/1299%0ARESEARCH

[39] Kahloun R, Jelliti B, Zaouali S, Attia S. Prevalence and causes of visual impairment in diabetic patients in Tunisia, North Africa. Eye. 2014;**28**(8): 986-991

[40] Ayukotang EN, Kumah DB, Mohammed AK. Prevalence of visual impairment among diabetic patients in the Kumba urban area, Cameroon. International Journal of Innovation and Applied Studies [Internet]. 2016;**15**(4): 872-876. Available from: http://www.ijias.issr-journals.org/

[41] Abejew AA, Belay AZ, Kerie MW. Diabetic complications among adult diabetic patients of a tertiary hospital in Northeast Ethiopia. Advances in Public Health Table [Internet]. 2015;**10**(1):1-8. DOI: 10.1155/2015/290920

[42] Bamashmus MA, Gunaid AA, Khandekar RB. Diabetic retinopathy, visual impairment and ocular status among patients with diabetes mellitus in

Yemen : A hospital-based study. Indian Journal of Ophthalmology. 2004;**57**(4): 293-298

[43] Chisha Y, Terefe W, Assefa H, Lakew S. Prevalence and factors associated with diabetic retinopathy among diabetic patients at Arbaminch General Hospital, Ethiopia: Cross sectional study. PLoS One. 2017;(3):1-9

[44] Cui Y, Zhang L, Zhang M, Yang X, Zhang L, Kuang J. Prevalence and causes of low vision and blindness in a Chinese population with type 2 diabetes. Scientific Reports [Internet]. 2017;7 (August):1-9. DOI: 10.1038/s41598-017-11365-z

[45] Cui Y, Zhang L, Zhang M, Yang X, Zhang L, Kuang J, Zhang G, Liu Q, HG & QM. Prevalence and causes of low vision and blindness in a Chinese population with type 2 diabetes. Sci Rep [Internet]. 2017;7(August):1-9. DOI: 10.1038/s41598-017-11365-z

[46] European Association for the Study of Obesity. International Obesity Task Force. Obesity. 2005;(March 15):1-9

[47] Colberg SR, Sigal RJ, Fernhall B, Regensteiner JG, Blissmer BJ, Rubin RR, et al. Exercise and type 2 diabetes: The American College of Sports Medicine and the American Diabetes Association: Joint position statement. Diabetes Care [Internet]. 2010;**33**(12):e150. Available from: care.diabetesjournals.org

[48] Bursac Z, Gauss CH, Williams DK, Hosmer DW. Source code for biology and purposeful selection of variables in logistic regression. bioMed Central [Internet]. 2008;**8**(17):1-8. Available from: http://www.scfbm.org/content/3/1/17

[49] Onakpoya OH, Kolawole BA, Adeoye AO, Adegbehingbe BO, Laoye O. Visual impairment and blindness in type 2 diabetics. International Ophthalmology. 2015;(Dm):1-9

[50] Zoungas S, Woodward M, Li Q, Cooper ME, Hamet P, Harrap S, et al. Impact of age, age at diagnosis and duration of diabetes on the risk of macrovascular and microvascular complications and death in type 2 diabetes. Diabetologia. 2014;**57**: 2465-2474

[51] Asano RY, Sales MM, Alberto R, Browne V, Fernando J, Nova V, et al. Acute effects of physical exercise in type 2 diabetes: A review. World Journal of disbetes [Internet]. 2014; **5**(5):659-665. Available from: https://www.researchgate.net/publication/264923848Acute

[52] Thent ZC, Das S, Henry LJ. Role of exercise in the management of diabetes mellitus : The global scenario. PLoS One. 2013;**8**(11):1-8

[53] Thomas D, Ej E, Ga N. Exercise for type 2 diabetes mellitus (Review). Cochrane Database Syst Rev [Internet]. 2009;(1):10–11. Available from: http://www.thecochrane library.com

[54] Yang D, Yang Y, Li Y, Han R. Physical exercise as therapy for type 2diabetes mellitus : From mechanism to orientation. Annals of Nutrition & Metabolism. 2019;**74**(295): 313-321

[55] Ababa A, Tekalegn Y, Addissie A, Kebede T, Ayele W. Magnitude of glycemic control and its associated factors among patients with type 2 diabetes at Tikur Anbessa specialized. PLUS ONE [Internet]. 2018; **13**(3):5-16. DOI: 10.1371/journal.pone.0193442

[56] Kim J, Kwon H, Park Y, Lee J, Kim M, Yoon K, et al. Prevalence and associated factors of diabetic retinopathy in Rural Korea. Journal of Korean Medical Science. 2011;**26**:1068-1073

[57] Wallace TM, Matthews DR. QJM Poor glycaemic control in type 2 diabetes : A conspiracy of disease, suboptimal therapy and attitude. The Quarterly Journal of Medicine. 2000;**93**:369-374